The
Marine Corps
3X
Fitness Program

THE
MARINE CORPS
3X
FITNESS PROGRAM

Martin Cohen

Little, Brown and Company
Boston/Toronto

FIRST EDITION

LIBRARY OF CONGRESS CATALOGING-IN-PUBLICATION DATA

Cohen, Martin Aver.
  The Marine Corps 3x fitness program.

  1. Physical fitness. 2. United States. Marine Corps. I. Title. II. Title:
Marine Corps three x fitness program.
GV481.C645 1986   613.7′1   85-18179
ISBN 0-316-15018-5
ISBN 0-316-15017-7 (pbk.)

All photographs by George Bennett

Before embarking on any strenuous exercise program, including the program described in this book, everyone, par-
ticularly anyone with any known heart or blood-pressure
problem, should be examined by a physician.

The views expressed in this book do not purport to reflect the
positions of the USMC, the Department of the Navy or the
Department of Defense.

BP

Published simultaneously in Canada
by Little, Brown & Company (Canada) Limited

PRINTED IN THE UNITED STATES OF AMERICA

For Knox Burger, Kitty Sprague,
and the legend

CONTENTS

Acknowledgments

THE author is indebted to many Marines for their help, including Brigadier General Gene A. Deegan, Colonel Robert H. Thompson, Lieutenant Colonel Robert E. Godwin, Lieutenant Colonel Robert J. Mastrion, Lieutenant Colonel John M. Shotwell, Major John D. Bratten, Major Richard C. Lepley, Major Patti Mauck, Major Wayne E. Rollins, Major Ron Stevens, Major James L. Vance, Captain Ralph Arquiette, Captain Gerald T. Janda, Captain William W. Miller, Captain Joanna Schilling, Captain Gary S. Supnick, First Lieutenant Jerry DeValle, First Lieutenant Michael F. Imsick, First Lieutenant Steve G. Manuel, First Lieutenant Rick L. Reece, Master Gunnery Sergeant William L. Dower (Ret.), Gunnery Sergeant Randall L. Bare, Gunnery Sergeant W. Vodaman Brown, Gunnery Sergeant R. M. Mayberry, Gunnery Sergeant Edward A. "Robbie" Roberts (Ret.), Gunnery Sergeant Judy Vina, Gunnery Sergeant Ernest W. Walter, Staff Sergeant Lorna M. Papke; and Color Sergeant G. H. Russell, Royal Marines, and Paul O. Davis, Institute of Human Performance.

In addition, the author wishes to thank the Marine Corps for permission to use material contributed by Marine Corps Headquarters, Washington, D.C., the Recruit Training Regiment and the Women's Training Command, Parris Island, South Carolina, the Officer Candidates School and The Basic School, Quantico, Virginia, the Physical Training Division, the Special Training Division and the Physical Fitness Center, Marine Corps Recruiting Depot, San Diego, California.

· 1 ·

The Elite Physique

THREE TOUGH QUESTIONS

BEFORE starting a conditioning program, you should ask the following questions:

Is the program practical and efficient?
What will it accomplish for me?
How do I know that it's good?
Here are the answers, the facts about Marine conditioning:

· The effectiveness of Marine conditioning is confirmed by the results. Of all the military services, the Marines are the fittest and trimmest, probably the best-conditioned men and women in the world.

· Marine conditioning is straightforward and easy to learn.

· Marine priorities are identical to the goals of civilians:

   1. A slender body and good posture because pride in appearance is a Marine tradition.

   2. The capacity for maximum performance on the job plus a reserve of stamina for personal activities and emergencies.

· Marine conditioning works for both men and women from age 18 to 55. Although the excellent condition of young, combat-ready Marines is to be expected, anyone visiting a Marine command is impressed by the superb appearance of all men and women, whether over or under 30, including administrative and clerical personnel whose workdays are comparable to civilians'.

· Marines are made, not born. Many enter the service with common civilian problems, including poor posture, excess body fat and insufficient energy to meet their daily responsibilities. As recruits, they develop elite fitness gradually and safely through modified conditioning, which is basic to the 3X Program. Using this procedure, even a sedentary civilian can enjoy quality fitness.

· Like a civilian, each Marine is personally responsible for maintaining fitness. The program requires no supervision, neither a platoon leader nor an exercise instructor.

· The 3X plan provides an essential lifetime fitness program whether you lead an athletic or sedentary life.

· Because Marines are stationed around the world, the 3X Program is designed for use in virtually any environment: in a city park or an embassy compound, in the confines of a small apartment or aboard a tight ship, and, when on the move, in a hotel or bunker.

· The Marine Corps has developed a method that measures the percentage of fat in the human body, a critical factor in achieving maximum performance, good health and a trim appearance. Part 4 of this book tells you how to assess the amount of fat that you carry and thus learn what percentage is best for you.

· The effectiveness of Marine conditioning is beyond question, verified at six-month intervals when commissioned and enlisted personnel, both men and women, undergo the Marine Physical Fitness Test. Part 3 tells you how to compare your fitness with Marine standards.

· Marine standards have maintained the Corps reputation as the nation's elite force for over 200 years. It is this concept of excellence that is available to you.

BASIC PRINCIPLES OF THE 3X PROGRAM

EVERY Marine, enlisted or commissioned, is personally responsible for maintaining a fitness program. This is not only a matter of practicing self-reliance, a Marine tradition, but is also based in sound exercise physiology. Extensive research tells us:

1. Individuals, including those in the same age group, test out at different levels of fitness. Therefore, most of us should begin conditioning at different levels.

2. Individuals also improve their fitness at different rates. As a result, a standardized program is counterproductive. If you are in an exercise class or work from a manual that prescribes the same number of repetitions for everyone, you are held back by the slowest person.

3. The inefficiency of a standardized program is further complicated because muscle groups improve at different rates. In an exercise class, for

example, you may be working at a level appropriate for your skeletal muscles but not vigorous enough for your cardiorespiratory system.

For these reasons, a sound, sophisticated conditioning program must adapt to the individual's starting level and capacity. This is true for everyone, including professional athletes as well as the men and women of the Marines. Although all Marines must ultimately meet the same physical standards, some advance rapidly, some at a moderate pace and others may require remedial workouts. And so, in a gym or outdoors, you will usually find a Marine working out alone.

The fitness of everyone, regardless of age or sex, improves at the individual's best pace, and that is another virtue of the 3X Fitness Program. These are some of its basic principles:

Progressive Conditioning

Understanding gradual conditioning is especially important to Marines and others who are highly motivated. People with strong drives, eager to shape up in a hurry, are likely to overdo a workout, which is not only inefficient but will likely bring on aches and possible injury. Therefore, it is important to understand that progressive conditioning is safe and practical.

Progressive conditioning is a continuous, gradual process. The continuum is basic in developing strength and endurance whether you are a recruit or a civilian who has been leading a sedentary life. If you look at the chart on page 6, you see that progressive conditioning is a simple upward line. No matter where you start on the line, and no matter how far you go, you must pass through each stage. It is impossible to leapfrog from any one point on the line to another.

The bottom of the line represents the minimum amount of fitness or conditioning that everyone must have to merely stay alive. A little more fitness represents the person who is just sitting up after a major injury. Suppose it is an Olympic athlete who has been flat on his back for weeks. On his first day out of bed he will need support because his skeletal muscles are weak. This illustrates the progressive principle in reverse: with disuse, muscles lose their tone. We all experience this to some degree.

For example, if you hibernate during the winter, your conditioning slides backward. It may be so gradual that you are unaware of what is happening. On the first day of spring, however, if you play tennis with a competitive friend or take a long hike into the woods, you may drop from exhaustion. And for several more days you will likely suffer the misery of sore muscles.

Still, your condition isn't any more hopeless than the convalescent's. With use, muscles strengthen. And so, day by day, as the patient makes an effort to walk a little longer, his muscles regain strength until he reaches the fitness

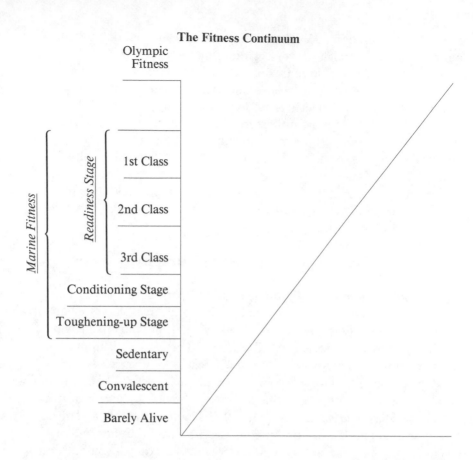

The Fitness Continuum

Olympic
Fitness

Marine Fitness

Readiness Stage

1st Class

2nd Class

3rd Class

Conditioning Stage

Toughening-up Stage

Sedentary

Convalescent

Barely Alive

level of the person who has been hibernating. Now he can handle work that requires a little physical exertion. On the chart, this stage is identified as the fitness level of the sedentary person, who is a major concern of health therapists, and with good reason.

Being sedentary means that you must always be sorry for yourself. When you run for a bus or train, your heart beats unmercifully and you gasp for breath. You have less resistance to common infections, and also lack the health to recover rapidly after an illness. You tire quickly during the day and sleep poorly at night. You are nagged by aches in the neck and lower back. And, unhappily, you are likely to be overweight.

Marine recruits reflect the fitness deficits of the sedentary population. A few may even be grossly overweight and underconditioned. In 10 to 12 weeks, however, recruits lose excess body fat and develop stamina and strength, but that is not accomplished with a crash program. That is the myth — that Marines are pushed to the breaking point, collapse, and then wake up the next morning with superhuman strength.

In fact, the making of a Marine is a deliberate, thoughtful procedure beginning with the recognition that conditioning must be progressive. The key to progressive conditioning is the overload principle.

The Overload Principle

To improve the condition of your body, an exercise must work your muscles and cardiorespiratory system a little harder than usual. This deliberate stressing of muscles during workouts is known as overloading. Between workouts, during recovery periods of 24 to 48 hours, the body goes through a rebuilding process. The muscles and the cardiorespiratory system become a little stronger and more efficient as the body prepares to meet new demands made by the overload.

The Comfort Index

A practical rule for progressive overloading is simple: when you feel comfortable during a workout, work a little harder. Many Marine men and women do this by making a maximum effort, which means trying for one, two or three more repetitions of an exercise after completing a routine workout. Not understanding the difference between exercising at a comfort level and making an extra effort results in frustration.

An example is the businessman who takes 25 minutes to walk the mile to his office. He complains that he feels no better and continues to be overweight. He believes this is proof that exercise does not work for him. His problem is misunderstanding the difference between exercise and conditioning exercise. His daily walk only maintains his fitness to repeat a leisurely walk.

If, however, the man decides to increase his daily walk to a mile and a half, and still do it in 25 minutes, he has put the overload principle to work. He will have to walk faster. As a result, his muscles must work harder and his cardiorespiratory system must deliver a little more oxygen than usual. He has gone beyond the comfort index, converting his daily walk into a conditioning exercise.

Instant Progress

The businessman's extra effort, which is the overload, instantly sets off a series of biological happenings that will result in improving his fitness. During the recovery period, the man's muscles, heart, lungs and vascular system respond to the demand by becoming stronger and more efficient. The man is now in the conditioning phase of a fitness program. During this phase, the individual has the option of using the overload principle to develop strength and endurance or only strength.

How You Develop Strength

Strength is defined as the measure of a muscle group when exerting maximum force. In Olympic competition, for example, the gold medal for strength goes to the person who is able to lift the heaviest weight just once. Strength is developed by lifting a weight, or performing a calisthenic, that you can at first repeat no more than 2 or 3 times. When you have worked up to about 8 repetitions, start over by increasing the workload. Because strength by itself has limited use in contemporary life, the Marines emphasize conditioning that develops both strength and endurance.

How You Develop Endurance

Muscular endurance is defined by physiologists as the ability to repeat an exercise many times or continue an activity for extended periods, and that is what Marines and civilians need most to get through the day successfully. Endurance gives us the energy to spend long hours at study and work, the exhilaration to enjoy leisure hours, and the stamina to practice and refine skills for skiing, tennis and other weekend sports. Endurance is developed with exercises that can be repeated at least 10 times but preferably 20 or more times.

There are 2 ways to go about developing endurance. One is to begin with an exercise that you can do only 2 or 3 times, for example, a pushup, and gradually develop the strength to perform 20 repetitions. This is inefficient because strength development is a slow process, and it will be a long time before you begin endurance conditioning.

The better way is to begin with an exercise that you can repeat about 10 times by lightening the workload. By modifying the pushup, for example, you reduce the amount of body weight to be lifted but retain the essential workout for upper-body muscles. In the 3X program, you will find 5 modifications of the pushup that are graded by the degree of overload. If you start with a modified version that you can repeat 10 times, you begin to develop endurance immediately. When you can perform 20 repetitions, move up to a slightly more demanding modification of the pushup, which further increases endurance.

Note that all these procedures depend on the overload principle. The benefits are extensive and specific. Overload conditioning helps prevent injuries such as sprains, strains and fractures; increases the ability to absorb shock and withstand stress, especially in the joints and joint connectors; and prevents or lessens the agony of backaches. Cardiovascular benefits include the development of many more capillaries, which improves the distribution of blood, thus increasing aerobic energy. Your heart will not have to work as hard under physical or mental stress whether you are running for a bus or adapting to the shock of bad news.

All of this leads to several questions:

How long do you continue overloading your body?

How much improvement do you need?

How much fitness do you need?

When do you level off and move into the maintenance level?

A PRIVATE MATTER

THE professional athlete, the Marine and the deskbound civilian are doing the same thing during the conditioning phase — all are overloading their muscles. Deciding when to discontinue overloading and go into the maintenance phase depends on individual needs. What these needs may be is found in the definition of physical fitness.

A physiologist defines physical fitness as the body's capacity to function in response to the demands of the environment. Glancing back at the illustration "The Fitness Continuum," we see that the degree of fitness ranges from the minimum needs of a person who is barely alive, perhaps in a coma, to the world-class demands of the Olympic competitor. Virtually no one needs as much conditioning as Olympic athletes, because their goal is shaving fractions of seconds off world records, and their conditioning is an exhausting, full-time occupation. For most of us, however, conditioning at high levels is a waste of time. We have no use for that much fitness — nor do the Marines, who are not in the business of producing athletes.

The Marine Corps defines fitness as readiness for maximum performance during the workday with a reserve capacity for emergencies, and this is similar to the goals of most civilians.

You can test your current fitness by Marine standards, which are listed by sex and age in Part 3. You may test yourself against minimum acceptable standards or, if you wish, take the challenge, as some Marines do, and shoot for higher scores. This is a private decision. Once the level of conditioning satisfies your needs, you move from a conditioning phase to a maintenance program.

THE GENERAL BENEFITS OF A MAINTENANCE PROGRAM

WHEN you follow a maintenance program, you can expect a number of physical and psychological benefits, including:

- Better health. You are less likely to become ill, but if you do, you will recover more quickly.
- Feeling better. Exercise releases hormones known as beta endorphins, natural, nonaddictive chemicals that relieve stress.
- The prevention of common injuries such as sprains and strains, and the elimination or lessening of backache.
- An increase of HDL's (high density lipoproteins). This results in the lowering of blood cholesterol, decreasing the risk of stroke and heart disease.
- More energy, more vigor and a zestier life.
- Increased lung and heart capacity. You will have a greater capacity for physical activity, whether it is dancing, sports, or merely the ability to walk briskly if you are late for an appointment.
- Better looks with the loss of excess body fat.
- Better looks because maintenance exercise helps maintain body weight at an attractive level.
- Better looks as muscles firm up.
- Better looks because muscle toning contributes to poise and good posture.
- Relief from daily tension because muscles relax after exercises. Furthermore, exercise produces sound sleep, which also produces a more relaxed state.

SPECIAL TREATMENT FOR WOMEN?

FITNESS tests for women are not as difficult as those for men because of biological differences. However, conditioning assures women dramatic improvement in all of their pursuits because excellence in performance depends on having the strength and endurance to use skills. Whether on the job or in weekend sports, a woman may develop the fitness to compete successfully with men.

Women should put effort into workouts and gradually increase their overload just as men do. Furthermore, and this is very important, exercises that work best for men are also best for women. A woman who fails to take advantage of these benefits is cheating herself of procedures that men commonly use to improve their appearance, health and energy.

SUMMING UP

CONDITIONING effectively improves the looks, performance and lives of everyone. Without reservation, the 3X Fitness Program is recommended in its entirety to both men and women.

·2·

The 3X Fitness Program

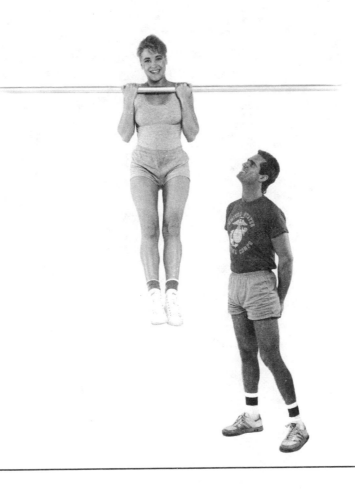

A FORMULA FOR EXCELLENCE

MARINE conditioning is a straightforward, goal-oriented program that produces the best in fitness for virtually anyone. It is based on the 3X formula, which is time-efficient and easy to learn.

3 Phases

Because conditioning should be progressive, the program falls into three divisions.

The Preparatory Phase. A toughening-up stage for the sedentary person or anyone out of condition because many of us tend to overdo workouts and suffer for it. For this reason, a preconditioning stage is built into the program. Beginning levels tone up your body safely and gradually to prepare you for the essential conditioning phase. Note: You may not have to go through the preparatory phase in every instance. For example, if you routinely take a brisk 30-minute walk, then you can begin cardiorespiratory conditioning at a walk/jog level.

The Conditioning Phase. This stage develops the conditioning power to meet Marine standards and your personal fitness goals. As explained earlier, Marines develop endurance as well as strength by executing a maximum number of repetitions. Power, the third goal, is achieved with high-speed contractions. During the conditioning phase, the emphasis is on performing as many repetitions as possible as rapidly as possible.

The Maintenance Phase. A program that maintains conditioning at a level compatible with your life-style because a fitness program should serve your needs.

3 Times a Week

Corps regulations state that each Marine is personally responsible for a minimum of three 1-hour workouts a week. Following this rule faithfully is critical to the maintenance of Marine excellence.

Only 3 Tests for Fitness

All 3X conditioning conforms to the physiologist's rule of specificity: to be effective, a conditioning plan must result in the body's adapting to specific standards. In the Marine program, standards have been established by 3 fitness tests, which evaluate the upper torso, lower torso, and cardiorespiratory system.

The 3-Cycle Workout

A procedure that guarantees substantial gains without punishment. Exercises, targeted at specific muscle groups, are cycled in sets of 3. The procedure is especially effective in overloading your body gradually.

3 Rules for Effective Conditioning

The following recommendations are essential to your health and progress.

Breathe Correctly: For safety's sake, learn to breathe properly to avoid feeling dizzy. Beginners often hold their breath during an intense workout, and this may cause faintness. To prevent such problems, develop the habit of breathing rhythmically while exercising. Practice exhaling during the part of the exercise that requires the most exertion. For example, when doing a situp, breathe out while raising your body, which is the intense part of the exercise. Inhale while lowering your body. Also note that you are most likely to breathe incorrectly during the last few repetitions of an exercise because these require the most effort.

Do It Right: Performing exercises haphazardly not only leads to strains and aches but also is a waste of energy. Good form, as important to exercise as it is to sports, produces the best results in the least time.

Pacing: In the beginning, work slowly until you can perform the exercise correctly. When your coordination is rhythmic and relaxed, increase your speed and the number of repetitions you execute. This will develop strength, endurance and power.

The remainder of this section will tell you how to put your program together.

THE EXERCISES: GETTING STARTED

BEGIN by selecting an exercise at a level that immediately begins to improve your endurance and strength. Do this by choosing the exercise in each classification that you can repeat about 10 times when making a maximum effort.

Lower-Body Conditioning: Choose 1 for Strength and Endurance

Purpose: Appearance is a priority with virtually everyone, and at the top of the list is doing something about a sagging midriff. This is accomplished by strengthening the hip flexors and abdominal muscles, which, in turn, flatten the stomach. Lower-torso conditioning also helps to overcome pelvic tilt and curvature of the spine by strengthening the pelvic girdle, and this helps prevent low back pain.

Furthermore, Marines find that lower-torso conditioning significantly improves coordination and endurance in any activity, whether it is walking, running, swimming or hurdling an obstacle course. Midriff conditioning provides the muscular support that is essential to tennis, golf, skiing and virtually all other sports. For these reasons, the lower torso is conditioned for endurance and strength.

The Exercise: The test that validates midriff and lower-torso fitness for men and women is the Marine situp. It also serves as the single, most dependable lifetime exercise to maintain a flat stomach and efficient posture. And that is why Marines routinely execute situps by the dozens.

THE MARINE SITUP AND ITS MODIFICATIONS

Do It Right: For the situp and all modifications, the starting position is the same: the supine position with your feet flat on the deck. The angle at your knees is about 45 degrees. Note that if your feet are too close to your thighs, the exercise becomes unnecessarily difficult.

Your feet, separated to the width of your shoulders, should be anchored under a bookcase, sofa, barbell or other heavy object. Action requires raising your upper body and bringing your head forward to your knees. Develop the habit of curling your body forward rather than snapping up, which may cause muscle strain. Breathe out on Count 1 as you raise yourself, breathe in during Count 2 as you return to the starting position.

Find Your Starting Level: The Marine situp has been modified to accommodate your present level of strength. Find the modification that you can repeat about 10 times when making a maximum effort. Enter your starting level in the chart on page 50.

Level 1: Sidearm Curl

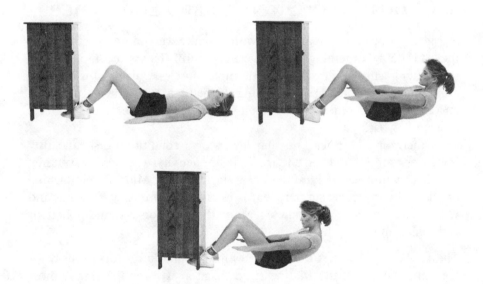

Starting Position: The supine position as described above.

Count 1: With arms along your sides, tuck your chin against your chest while curling your body forward. To maintain balance, let your arms rise parallel to the deck. Continue curling forward until your shoulders are about 10 inches off the deck, or until you see the tops of your knees.

Count 2: Return to starting position.

Tempo: Start slowly and work up to your best speed.

Goal: Execute maximum number of repetitions at each workout. When you can perform 20 continuous repetitions, move on to Level 2.

Level 2: Hip Curl

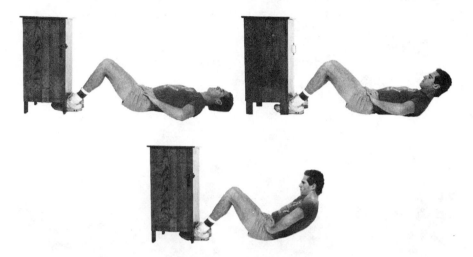

Starting Position: Same as above with hands on hips. Two counts same as above but hands remain on hips.

Tempo: Start slowly and work up to your best speed.

Goal: Execute maximum number of repetitions at each workout. When you can perform 20 continuous repetitions, move on to Level 3.

Level 3: Head Curl

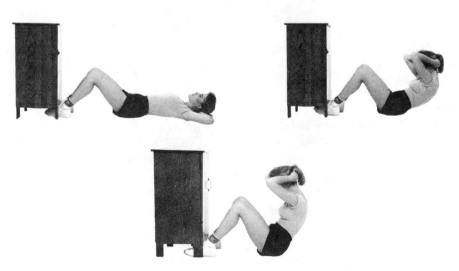

Starting Position: Same as above with fingers laced behind head. Two counts same as above but hands remain locked behind head.

Tempo: Start slowly and work up to your best speed.

Goal: Execute maximum number of repetitions at each workout. When you can perform 20 continuous repetitions, move on to Level 4.

Level 4: Sidearm Situp

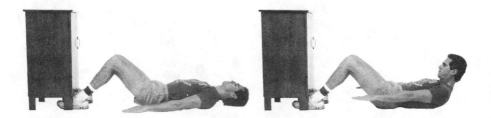

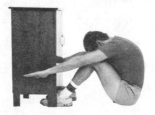

Starting Position: Same as above with arms along sides.

Count 1:   Sit up, curling your head as far forward as possible. As you get better at this, your head will break an imaginary plane between your knees. Do not use either your hands or arms for support. As you curl forward, your arms will rise alongside your body, parallel to the deck. The arms are used only for balance, because your abdominal muscles are doing most of the work.

Count 2:   Return to supine starting position.

Tempo: Start slowly and work up to your best speed.

Goal: Execute maximum number of repetitions at each workout. When you can perform 20 continuous repetitions, move on to Level 5.

Level 5: Hip Situp

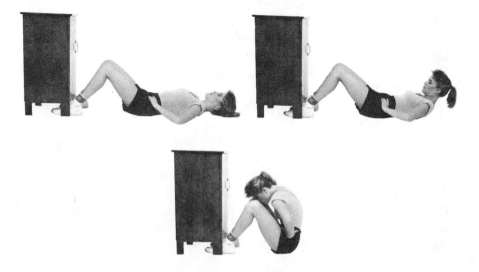

Starting Position: Same as above with hands on hips. Two counts same as the above with hands on hips.
Tempo: Start slowly and work up to your best speed.
Goal: Execute maximum number of repetitions at each workout. When you can perform 20 continuous repetitions, move on to Level 6.

Level 6: The Marine Situp

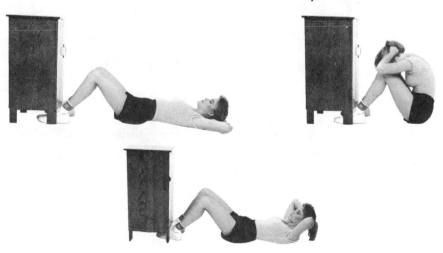

Starting Position: With your feet flat on the deck and your knees flexed, take the supine position. Your shoulder blades are touching the deck, your hands clasped behind your head. Anchor your feet under a radiator, water pipe, sofa, large chair, bookcase or any other stationary object. Or someone may hold your feet or legs below your knees.

Count 1: Raise upper body, curling forward until your face breaks an imaginary plane through the knees.

Count 2: Lower trunk to starting position. Note that shoulder blades must touch the deck to complete each repetition. During the entire movement, your hands are clasped behind your head, and your feet must remain anchored to the deck.

Tempo: Start slowly and work up to your best speed.

Goal: Continue until you can execute 20 or more situps. The sky is the limit. When you can perform over a 100, you may shoot the moon. Increase the overload by elevating your feet. Begin with a low object, such as a footstool or coffee table, then gradually increase the overload, placing your feet on higher objects such as a sofa, chair, table and, finally, a high stool as photographed.

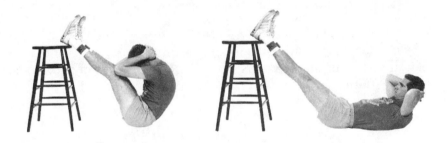

Upper-Body Conditioning: Choose 3 for Endurance and Strength

Purpose: Although most of us worry about our waistline, studies find that our upper torso — shoulders, arms and chest — suffers the most neglect. Tests of Marine recruits, who reflect civilian problems, find that a man may not be able to do a single pullup; a woman not one pushup. This is unfortunate.

Upper-torso conditioning is essential to the prevention of fatigue whether the activity is administrative or domestic, carrying responsibility or a bag of groceries, competing in the executive suite or on the tennis court. Furthermore, upper-body strength is basic to good posture, good looks and the prevention of low back pain.

The Exercises: Marines depend on several exercises to overcome upper-torso weakness. The most reliable include the pushup, the triceps dip, the pullup and the flexed-arm hang, or modifications of these exercises.

The pushup, a mainstay in maintaining Marine fitness, can be performed anywhere — alongside a bed or desk, or in the aisle of a transport plane.

THE PUSHUP AND ITS MODIFICATIONS

Do It Right: In the starting position, feet and legs should be parallel. Hands should be about shoulder-distance apart with fingers pointed forward, and palms flat against the wall, the deck or other surface. Most important, whether doing a pushoff or pushup, your back and legs should remain straight throughout the exercise. Exhale when pushing; inhale on the return.

Find Your Starting Level: Test your upper fitness among the following modifications of the pushup. The version that you can repeat about 10 times, when making a maximum effort, is your starting level. Enter it in the chart on page 50.

Level 1: Wall Pushoff

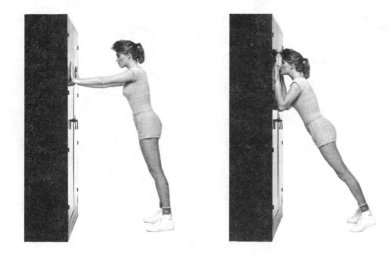

Starting Position: Step back a distance of 2 to 3 feet from a wall. Place your hands against the wall at shoulder level. Now lean into the wall, keeping your arms straight and your elbows locked. Your arms should be supporting the weight of your upper body because you will, in effect, be doing a vertical pushup.

Count 1: Bend elbows outward, bringing your body forward until your nose touches the wall.

Count 2: Push back to starting position to complete 1 repetition.

Tempo: Start slowly and work up to your best speed.

Goal: When you can perform 20 continuous repetitions, move on to Level 2.

Level 2: Chest-High Pushoff

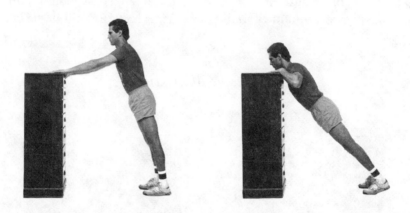

Starting Position: Choose a piece of furniture that stands as high as your chest, such as a piano, chest of drawers or bookcase. Take the pushoff/ pushup position described above, with your hands placed firmly on the top side of the furniture. Your body should be straight, inclined like a board. Your body weight is now resting on your hands and the balls of your feet.

Count 1: Bending elbows outward, lower your body until your chest barely touches the surface.

Count 2: Push back to starting position to complete one repetition.

Tempo: Start slowly and work up to your best speed.

Goal: When you can perform 20 continuous repetitions, move on to Level 3.

Level 3: Waist-High Pushoff

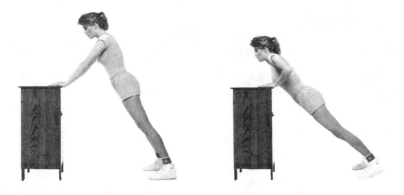

Starting Position: Same as above, pushing off a waist-high surface such as a table or desk.
Goal: When you can perform 20 continuous repetitions, move on to Level 4.

Level 4: Knee-High Pushoff

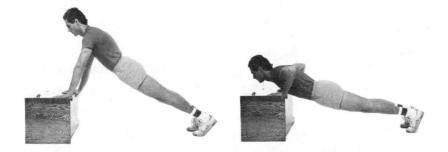

Starting Position: Same as above, using a bed, sofa, bench or other surface that is about knee high.
Goal: When you can perform 20 continuous repetitions, move on to Level 5.

Level 5: Partial Pushup

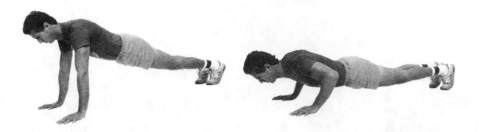

Starting Position: Take the prone position on the deck or on level ground. Hands are shoulder-distance apart, flat on the surface and pointed forward. Your body is totally supported by your hands and by the toes and balls of your feet. Your arms should be straight with elbows locked. Legs are also straight with feet together.

Count 1:   Bending elbows outward, lower your body until your chin is about 4 inches from the deck.

Count 2:   Push up to starting position to complete 1 repetition.

Tempo: Begin slowly, checking to be sure that your body is in a plane from your feet to your head. Gradually work up to your best speed.

Goal: When you can perform 20 continuous repetitions, move on to Level 6.

Level 6: The Marine Pushup

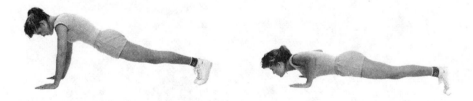

Starting Position: Take the prone position on the deck or on level ground. Your hands, shoulder-distance apart, are flat on the surface and pointed forward. Your body is supported by your hands and the balls of your feet. Arms should be straight with elbows locked. Legs are also straight with knees and feet together.

Count 1:   Bending elbows outward, lower your body until your chest just touches the deck. Remember that your chest must touch the deck during each repetition.

Count 2: Return to starting position.

Tempo: Begin slowly, checking yourself to be sure that your body is in a plane from your feet to your head. Gradually increase pace to your best speed.

Goal: When you can execute 80 or more repetitions continuously, you may shoot the moon with any of the following methods to perform advanced pushups:

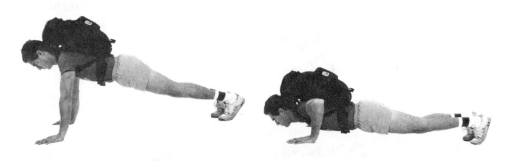

Method 1: To increase the body load, strap on a knapsack or backpack weighted with books and magazines. Start off with 10 to 15 pounds. When you can perform 20 continuous repetitions, add another 5 to 10 pounds. Within reason, and depending on your goal, you may pack the bag with additional weight as your strength increases.

Method 2: Continue to perform Marine pushups with your hands placed on the deck but increase the body load by elevating your feet on a box or carton that is 6 to 9 inches high. When you can perform 20 continuous repetitions, raise your feet slightly higher, perhaps to the edge of a bunk or the seat of a chair. When you are ready to increase the load again, place your feet on a table or desk. To further increase the load, strap a weighted knapsack to your back. Remember, however, that no matter how high your feet are elevated, your body must be kept straight from heels to head while exercising.

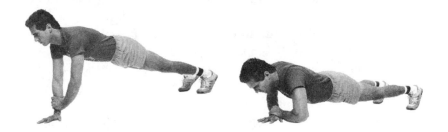

Method 3: Perform one-arm pushups as demonstrated in pictures.

Conditioning the triceps, the large muscles that run along the back of the upper arm, is essential to the development of arm strength as well as the firming of backside flesh that often annoys women. The exercise commonly used by Marines for these purposes is the triceps dip.

Do It Right: In the triceps dip and its modifications, your feet are together, your legs straight, arms along your sides. Hands, used for support, are pointed forward. Inhale while lowering yourself, exhale when raising your body.

Find Your Starting Level: Find the modification that you can repeat about 10 times when making a maximum effort. This is your starting level. Enter it in the chart on page 50.

Level 1: Sitdown Dips

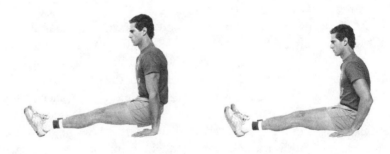

Starting Position: Take the sitting position on ground or deck with legs extended and feet together. Hands are flat on the deck, alongside your buttocks. Arms are straight with elbows locked, thus lifting your buttocks off the deck. You are now solely supported by your heels and hands.

Count 1: Bend your arms, lowering yourself until your buttocks touch the deck.

Count 2: Return to starting position.

Tempo: Start slowly, increasing your pace as you develop strength and coordination.

Goal: When you test out with 20 continuous repetitions, go on to Level 2.

Level 2: Off-the-Block Dips

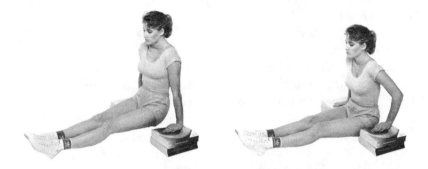

Same as Level 1 with your hands supported on blocks, boxes, telephone directories or any other objects that raise your buttocks about 12 inches off the deck.

Goal: When you test out with 20 continuous repetitions, go on to Level 3.

Level 3: Off-the-Bench (or Sofa) Dips

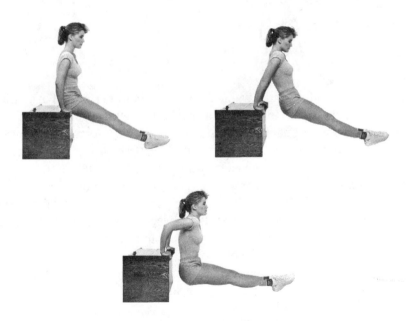

Starting Position: Sit on the edge of a stationary bench, coffee table, bed or sofa and grip the edge with both hands. Straighten your legs, locking your knees. Then straighten your arms, lifting your buttocks forward and off the edge of the surface. Your elbows should be locked, arms along your sides, with your body suspended and supported only by your hands and feet. This is your starting position.

Count 1: Bend your elbows to lower your buttocks below the edge of the stationary surface.

Count 2: Push up to starting position to complete one repetition.

Goal: When you can perform 20 continuous repetitions go on to Level 4. Otherwise, continue with modified dips, increasing your pace and number of repetitions. You can also increase the overload of modified dips by elevating your feet on a stool or chair, or by strapping a weight to your back.

Level 4: Standard and Advanced Triceps Dips

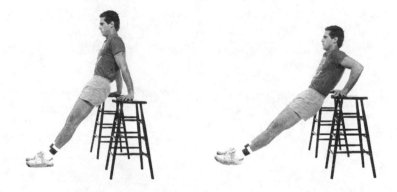

Equipment: Standard and advanced dips are usually performed in gymnasiums on parallel bars. However, Marines in the field are often driven by necessity to find a reasonable substitute for parallel bars. As a result, they use a variety of props, ranging from a staircase or tree stump to a fence or concrete wall. In the following exercises, high wooden stools (with rubber feet to prevent dangerous slips) serve as substitutes for parallel bars.

Starting Position: Hands are firmly set on stools with arms straight. Buttocks are suspended between the stools with legs stretched forward and feet on deck. Arms support the upper body while your feet partially support your lower body, thus modifying the overload.

Count 1: Bending arms at elbows, lower your body until your hands are alongside your rib cage, about 6 inches below your armpits.

Count 2: Return to starting position.

Tempo: Work at a comfortable pace, increasing your rhythm as you develop strength and coordination.

Goal: When you can perform 20 continuous repetitions, go on to Level 5.

Level 5: Bent-Knee Dips

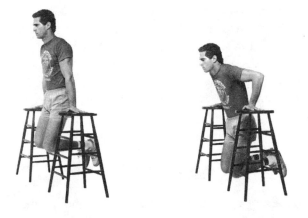

Equipment: Same as above.

Starting Position: Hands are firmly set on stools with arms straight. Knees are bent, thus suspending your body between the stools. Your arms support all of your body weight.

Count 1: Bend your elbows, lowering your body until your hands are alongside your rib cage.

Count 2: Return to starting position.

Tempo: Work at a comfortable pace, increasing your rhythm as you develop strength and coordination.

Goal: When you can perform 20 continuous repetitions, go on to Level 6.

Level 6: Pike Dips

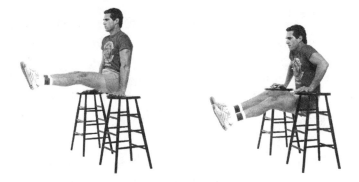

Equipment: Same as above.

Starting Position: Same as above with legs extended parallel in the pike position. Your arms are straight, supporting all of your body weight.

Count 1: Bend your elbows, lowering your body until your hands are alongside your rib cage.

Count 2: Return to starting position.

Note: You may increase the overload of any of the above by adding a back weight as explained in advanced pushups (see page 27).

Tempo: Work at a comfortable pace, increasing your pace as your coordination and strength increases.

Goal: 20 or more continuous repetitions.

PULLUPS/CHINUPS AND THE FLEXED-ARM HANG

As a primary test of upper-body fitness, the Marines require that both men and women demonstrate their ability to manage their own body weight. The tests are simple: for women, the flexed-arm hang, for men, either the pullup or chinup. The results, when recruits are tested, may be surprising.

A woman recruit who thinks of herself as a credible athlete discovers that she can barely hang on to the bar. And though the pullup may appear to be an ordinary test of conditioning, a husky male recruit may be lucky to do one. The problem is that few of us engage in activities that condition our upper bodies. A direct solution, the Marines have learned, is using the tests, the pullups and flexed-arm hangs, as conditioning exercises.

Besides developing shoulder-girdle strength and endurance, the benefits of pullups and the flexed-arm hang include increased grip strength, which pays off with better performance in sports that require racquets and bats, and the firming of jaw and throat muscles to improve appearance. Still, for the person who cannot do a single pullup, getting started appears to be insurmountable. It isn't.

The Marines, traditionally resourceful, have come up with exercises that develop strength for a difficult exercise by simulating movements that use the same muscles. One proven method of making an exercise practical is to reduce the body weight you must lift. An example is the Marine wounded in combat and hospitalized for a lengthy period. When he began to think about reconditioning his upper torso, he practiced modified pullups with a hospital trapeze while lying on his back. Although his muscles had partly atrophied from disuse, he was able to work his muscles through the motions of a standard chinup because he was lifting only part of his body weight.

A slightly different approach to reducing body weight is commonly used by parents. If a youngster cannot pull himself over a fence, the parent helps with a little boost, reducing the amount of body weight the child must lift.

Similarly, at recruit training depots, the Marines use a contraption that looks a little like a sling. This supports part of the body weight and allows the recruit to execute modified pullups.

The reverse calisthenic is another method of developing strength for a difficult exercise. In the reverse chinup or pullup, for example, you eliminate the difficult step, which is pulling yourself up to the bar. Instead, you step up on a box or stool and start the exercise in the chinning position. You then lower your body as slowly as possible until your arms are straight and immediately drop to the deck. Using the stool, you step up again to the starting position. This reverse, one-count exercise has the advantage of putting your muscles through the pullups full range of movement.

Any man or woman can develop strength for pullups and chinups using these modifications. However, to avoid frustrating yourself by expecting too much too soon, keep in mind that the pullup or chinup is a strength exercise in which you are attempting to lift your entire body weight. If you were lifting a barbell that weighed as much, you would expect it to be difficult.

Remember, too, that we develop strength by working with a weight so heavy that we can only manage a few repetitions. Although it may take a great effort to do only 1 or 2 pullups, you are making real progress. Developing strength by as much as 50%, for example going from 2 to 3 pullups, takes several times as long as tripling endurance, to go from 5 to 15 pushups. Although strength exercises require patience, there is an advantage: the workout takes less time.

Men and women may choose the modification that reduces body weight or the reverse calisthenic. Marines offer women the additional option of choosing the flexed-arm hang as an upper-body conditioner.

Important: When exercise bars are not available, Marines continue upper-body conditioning with pushups and modified triceps dips. On page 52, you will find 3-cycle workouts that do not include pullups and flexed-arm hangs.

THE PULLUP/CHINUP AND ITS MODIFICATIONS

Equipment: Horizontal chinning bar.

Do It Right: Chinning the bar means raising your body until your chin is above the bar on the first count, and then lowering your body until your arms are fully extended on the second count. Marines may choose between the chinup and pullup. The exercises differ only in the grip: palms face outward when executing the chinup; inward for the pullup. The pullup is a little easier. Exhale when chinning; inhale while lowering your body.

Find Your Starting Level: Because the pullup or the chinup is primarily a strength exercise, begin with a modified exercise that you can repeat no more than 3 times. Enter your starting level in the chart on page 50. Note that the exercises below may be further modified with a reverse pullup/chinup.

Level 1: Chest-High Pullup

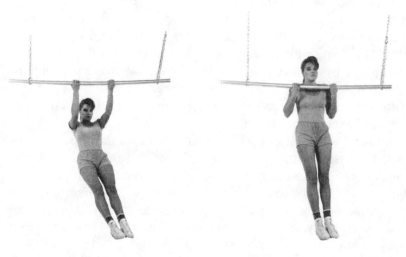

Starting Position: Secure horizontal bar at chest level. Grasp the bar with palms facing you. Slide your feet forward until your arms are fully extended. Your legs should be fairly straight. Your feet support the lower body throughout the exercise.
Count 1: Pull up until your chin is just over the bar but not touching it.
Count 2: Return to starting position.
Tempo: Exercise at a pace that allows you to make a maximum effort.
Goal: When you can chin the bar 10 times, move on to the next level.

Level 2: Chin-High Pullup

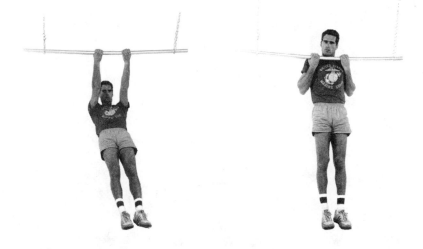

Same as Level 1 with the bar raised to chin height.

Level 3: Extended-Arm Pullup/Chinup

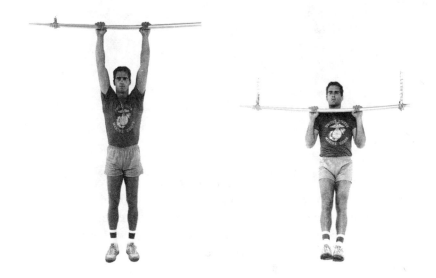

Starting Position: Raise the bar to a level that you can reach when you are standing upright and your feet are flat on the deck.

Count 1:   Pull up as high as possible, rising onto your toes, and then lift your feet off the deck.
Count 2:   Return to starting position.
Tempo: Your option.
Goal: When you can chin yourself 6 to 9 times, move on to Level 4.

Level 4: Partial Pullup/Chinup

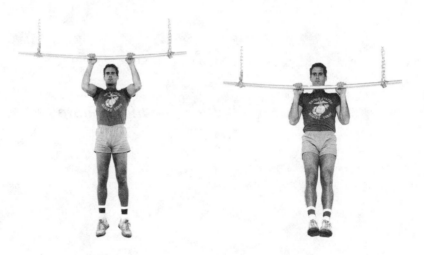

Starting Position: Raise horizontal bar beyond your reach. Throughout this exercise your body will be completely suspended. In the starting position, your legs will be fully extended but your arms are bent at the elbows to about a 45-degree angle. (See picture.) You may get into position with the assistance of a companion, box or stool.
Count 1:   Pull up your body until your chin is slightly above the bar.
Count 2:   Lower yourself to the starting position.
Tempo: Your option.
Goal: When you can perform 10 repetitions, move on to Level 5.

Level 5: The Marine Pullup/Chinup

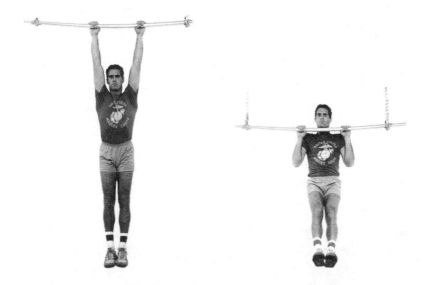

Starting Position: Grasp the bar with both hands. Your body is stretched out, your arms and legs fully extended and your feet off the deck.

Count 1: Keep your elbows along your sides while raising your body. You may kick your legs, if necessary, but not to the extent that your body swings. You complete the first count when your chin is above the bar. If you wish, you may rest in this position but your chin may not touch the bar.

Count 2: Return to the hanging position with your feet still free of the deck. You may rest in this position if you wish.

Tempo: Optional.

Goal: As many as possible. Three or more is good. Seven or more is very good. Twenty consecutive pullups earns a score of 100 in the fitness test. Again, note that patience is the key to developing pullups and chinups.

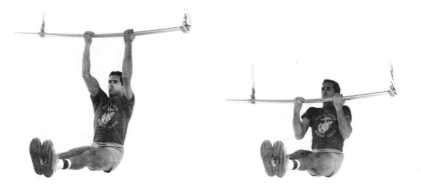

When it's easy to execute 20 chinups, shoot the moon. Wear a weighted backpack. Or execute chinups in the pike position, which means holding your legs at a right angle to your body. (See photographs on page 37.) To further increase the challenge, perform pike chinups with a weighted backpack.

When you have a fixed horizontal bar at a height that requires you to start conditioning at Level 4, which may be too difficult, begin with reverse pullups.

THE REVERSE PULLUP

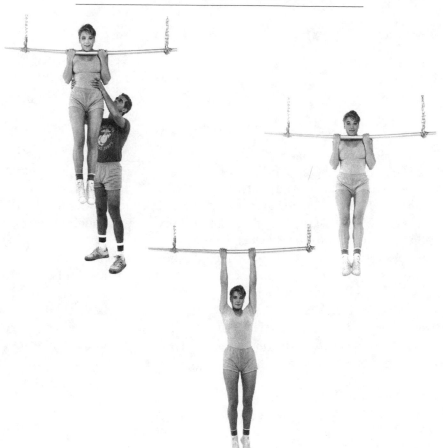

The reverse pullup is recommended to the underconditioned beginner. It will help virtually anyone develop the muscle to execute the classic chinup. *Starting Position:* Your partner may boost you, or you may use a box or stool to reach the horizontal bar. Grasp the bar with both hands, palms facing inward. Next, bend your elbows to position your chin slightly above the bar.

When your grip is firm, hang free maintaining flexion.

Count 1: From the flexed-arm position gradually lower yourself until your body is stretched out.

Count 2: Drop to the deck, step up to the bar and repeat first count.

Tempo: Optional.

Goal: When you can repeat the exercise up to 20 times, try the partial pullup, Level 4.

Note: You may also do this as a reverse chinup, grasping the bar with an overhand grip.

THE FLEXED-ARM HANG AND A MODIFICATION

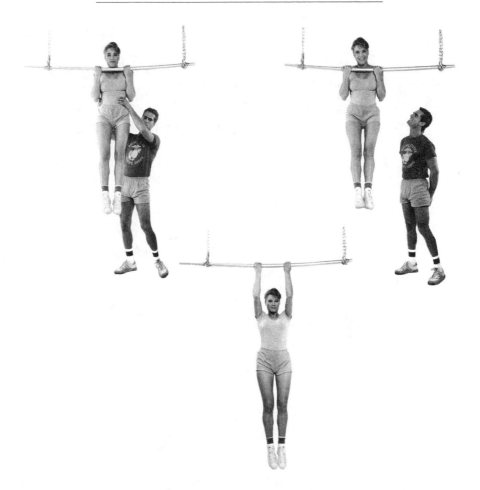

The flexed-arm hang is the Marine woman's test of upper-body fitness. (See Part 3: The Marine Physical Fitness Test.) The hang is also commonly used by Marine women as an exercise. For the flexed-arm hang, the horizontal bar is placed high enough that the woman's legs, when fully extended, do not touch the deck.

Starting Position: You may have a boost from a companion or use a box to step up to the bar. Grasp the bar with both hands, palms facing inward. Then bend your elbows to position your chin slightly above the bar. When your grip is firm, step off the box and let your body hang free. Note that you are not permitted to rest your chin on the bar at any time.

Count 1:   Maintain flexion in your elbows as long as possible. Time yourself by counting off the seconds in your head or on the wall clock. Some Marine women silently recite the Lord's Prayer or the lyrics of a song. Remember to continue timing yourself as long as you have any degree of flexion in your elbows.

Count 2:   When your arms are straight, immediately stop timing yourself, and drop to the deck.

Goal: To maintain flexion in the elbows as long as possible. If the flexed-arm hang is too difficult, begin with the modified hang.

THE MODIFIED FLEXED-ARM HANG

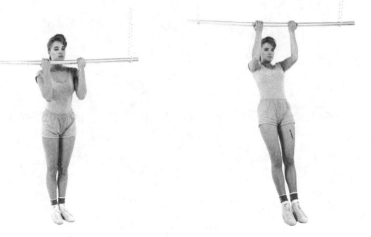

Same as the flexed-arm hang except that the horizontal bar is secured at shoulder- or chest-high level. When you are in the flexed-arm position, move your feet forward until your legs are straight and your lower torso is supported by your feet. When you can support yourself in the modified position for a minute, step up to the flexed-arm hang.

Note: Because the flexed-arm hang is an isometric exercise, it may be to your advantage to substitute a motion exercise such as a modified or reverse pullup, and then use the flexed-arm hang to test your progress.

Cautionary Note: In motion exercises, when muscles are continuously contracting and relaxing, there is no interference with blood circulation. In an isometric exercise, however, muscles are immobilized, in static contraction. This constricts blood vessels and may raise a person's blood pressure. People with hypertension, although usually encouraged to exercise, are cautioned to avoid isometric exercises such as the flexed-arm hang.

Cardiorespiratory Conditioning, Hip and Leg Toning, and Weight Control: Choose 1

Purpose: To improve cardiorespiratory efficiency. This results in the savings of thousands of heartbeats, or pumping actions, each day, which increases vigor and the capacity to function under stress. To burn off body fat and maintain desirable body weight. To enjoy other benefits, including increased productivity, restful sleep and better health. In addition, cardiorespiratory exercises improve flexibility, coordination, agility, balance, strength and endurance.

Cardiorespiratory fitness has the highest priority in Marine conditioning because of its unique contribution to performance, survival and the quality of life. No one remains a Marine unless he or she maintains a high level of cardiorespiratory efficiency.

THE WALK/JOG/RUN PROGRAM

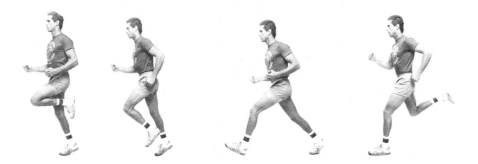

Exercise: Cardiorespiratory conditioning requires an exercise that increases the heartbeat substantially. This calls for sustained, rhythmic movement of the legs and the arms in such activities as running, walking, rope jumping and swimming. The Corps primary workout is walk/jog/run.

Do It Right: Poor running posture, such as stooping or leaning forward, strains the back. When running correctly, your head will be up and your body upright. This is when situps pay off and you discover that abdominal conditioning is the key to good posture.

The skeletal muscles of the upper body should be fairly relaxed. Elbows are flexed with arms swinging easily along the sides of your body, not across your chest; hands are cupped in a thumbs-up position but not clenched. Your head and neck are also relaxed. If your head tends to bobble, this can be corrected by gazing at a fixed object on the horizon.

Good locomotion depends on moving your legs with strength and coordination. Viewed in slow motion, a knee raises and then the leg stretches forward while you push off with the other leg. If, however, you merely kick your legs backward and forward, the calf muscles may be strained. Instead of taking small steps, get in the habit of stretching your pace.

Toes should not point out. To determine if your feet are hitting the ground parallel and in a straight line, stop running for a moment and check yourself with a knee bend. Bend slowly. If you are placing your feet properly, your knees will point directly ahead. If, however, you find that you are running with your feet turned out, it may be worthwhile to toe in a little in order to establish a correct habit. Finally, run off the whole of your foot, heel to toes. These recommendations are critical in preventing injuries to feet, knees, hips and back.

Take your time in learning good form. Think about the way you place your feet and move your legs, and keep your head and eyes up. After a while, walking and running correctly will become a lifetime habit, and it's to your advantage. Besides helping to prevent strains and sprains, good form is rewarded with better running time.

Practice relaxed breathing. Begin your workouts by shaking the tension out of your shoulders. Let your arms swing easily. As your pace quickens and your body demands more oxygen, you will breathe through your mouth. This is normal. Continue, however, to relax your arms and upper torso. This helps to conserve energy and strength.

Try to avoid running on hard surfaces that may overstress the legs. Also try to keep away from heavy traffic to avoid fumes and accidents. When possible, run in the cool of the day, and wear loose, porous clothes.

Progression: The principle of progression applies to cardiorespiratory conditioning just as it does to skeletal muscles. By gradually increasing the demand made on your lungs, heart and vascular system, the cardiorespiratory system improves. This is accomplished by overloading the cardiorespiratory system for a minimum of 30 minutes. You do this with a vigorous workout, but what is vigorous depends on your current state of fitness.

For example, if you can walk comfortably at a fast pace, then you will have to increase the overload by alternating jogging and walking. When you are comfortable with the walk/jog mode, you must jog more than you walk, and, eventually, run more than you jog to work at a vigorous level.

With progress, you will discover that you breathe easier when you run or walk briskly. Although your pulse rate rises during a workout, your heart will not be pounding. Furthermore, you will recover your normal pulse rate sooner after the workout.

Find Your Starting Level: The rate of progress in cardiorespiratory conditioning differs so much from one person to another that the Marines recommend individual training. For this reason, the Walk/Jog/Run plan has been modified to accommodate your present cardiorespiratory condition, whether you are unusually active or lead a sedentary life.

Marines seldom use a pulse reading during workouts. Instead, conditioning is direct and uncomplicated. At preparatory levels, the goal is sustaining a vigorous workout for 10 or more minutes. With cardiorespiratory improvement, three factors are added: speed, time and distance. The principal goal, however, is developing the capacity to sustain vigorous cardiorespiratory workouts for 30 or more minutes. It is that simple.

The key to safe, gradual conditioning is alternating between the work mode and the recovery mode. The workouts are expressly titled "Walk/Jog/Run" because you always have the option of dropping back to a walking or jogging gait. If you are feeling lightheaded or exhausted, immediately reduce your pace until your breathing and heartbeat return to a normal level.

Find your starting level below and enter it in the chart on page 50.

Level 1: Walk-Before-You-Jog

Purpose: A preconditioning phase for the sedentary person or anyone who has been hibernating or ill. Although this level is limited to walking, note that the session alternates between a work mode and a recovery mode.

Work Mode: Walk at a moderate to brisk pace. If you begin to feel excessively fatigued or winded, go to the recovery mode.

Recovery Mode: Walk at an easy pace or rest until you are breathing comfortably, then return to the work mode.

Workout: Continue alternating the work and recovery modes for three 10-minute periods as part of the 3X Conditioning Cycle. See page 48.

Goal: When you can maintain a vigorous walk for three 10-minute periods or 30 continuous minutes, go to Level 2.

Level 2: Walk 50/Jog 50

Purpose: To make the transition from walking to jogging. Warm up with a vigorous walk and then alternate the following modes.
Work Mode: Jog 50 paces.
Recovery Mode: Walk 50 paces.
Workout: Continue alternating the work and recovery modes for three 10-minute periods as part of the 3X Conditioning Cycle. See page 48.
Note: When you begin Level 2, you may not be able to alternate a 50-step jog for a full 10-minute workout. Do your best. If at any time you feel excessively fatigued, rest or, preferably, work out the remaining time walking at a comfortable pace.
Goal: When you can alternate 50 paces of jogging and walking continuously for 10 minutes, go to Level 3.

Level 3: Add-a-Minute Jog/Walk

Purpose: To continue gradual, safe cardiorespiratory conditioning. This is accomplished by increasing the intensity 1 minute at a time during the work mode.
Work Mode: Jog 2 minutes and then go into the recovery mode.
Recovery Mode: Walk about 50 paces until your breathing is comfortable, then return to the work mode.
Workout: Continue alternating the work and recovery modes for three 10-minute periods as part of the 3X Conditioning Cycle. See page 48.
Goal: When you can jog with reasonable comfort for 2 consecutive minutes, increase your jogging time to 3 minutes. Note that the Marine progression rule is in effect. Whenever you can complete the jogging period without special effort or incurring excessive fatigue, add another minute to the work mode. When you can jog 10 minutes continuously, move on to Level 4.

Level 4: The 11-Minute Mile

Purpose: To make the transition from jogging to running, and to prepare for the Marine cardiorespiratory test, which is based on time and distance.
Work Mode: After you have warmed up to your usual jogging gait, stretch

out your legs a bit. When the longer stride becomes comfortable, run slightly faster by pushing a little more on the rear leg.

Recovery Mode: If you become winded or excessively fatigued, drop back to a jog or walk. Remain at a recovery pace until you are no longer over-breathing, and then return to the work mode.

Goal: When you can run a measured mile comfortably in 11 minutes, move on to the next level.

Level 5: The 10-Minute Mile

Same as Level 4 until you can run/walk 1 mile in 10 minutes.

Level 6: The 1.5-Mile Run/Walk

Same as above until you can run/walk 1.5 miles in 15 to 18 minutes.

Level 7: The 2-Mile Run/Walk

Same as above until you can run/walk 2 miles in 20 to 23 minutes.

Level 8: The 2.5-Mile Run/Walk

Same as above until you can run/walk 2.5 miles in 24 to 27 minutes.

Level 9: The 3-Mile Run/Walk

Same as above until you can run/walk 3 miles in 28 to 30 minutes.

Your rate of progress depends on several factors, including your age, sex, weight and your current state of fitness. If you find that you have moved along too fast, or perhaps find that a higher level is exhausting, give yourself a little more time at the preceding level. Men and women, especially those 45 and over, should have the approval of a physician, preferably a cardiologist, before working toward Marine standards.

Alternate Cardiorespiratory Workouts

Other cardiorespiratory workouts are not merely optional but often a necessity. The person with blisters or a bad back may not be able to run, but can get comparable conditioning with cycling or swimming. And if bad weather or other factors keep you indoors, other useful substitutes include the boxer's rope jump and the stationary run. The following alternatives are productive in developing and maintaining cardiorespiratory fitness.

Walk/Run-in-Place:

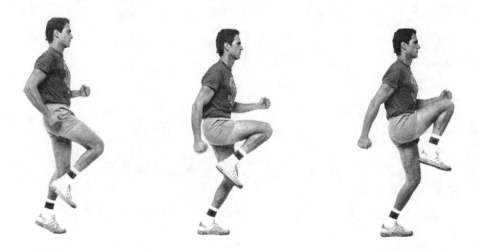

Marines commonly use the stationary run during a warmup drill, in a small gymnasium or aboard a ship. When you substitute walk/run-in-place for running, follow the progressive schedule laid out in the walk/jog/run plan. If indoors, run-in-place on a mat or thick carpet, and wear running shoes to lessen stress. Note that the pumping action of your arms also increases your heartbeat. While exercising, keep your arms in motion and lift your feet about 8 inches. Your knees will rise to about the level of your hips. As your conditioning improves, gradually raise your knees to waist level.

Rope Jump:

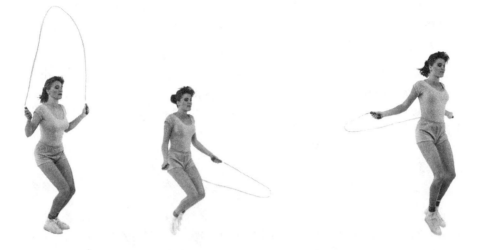

This is an excellent cardiorespiratory exercise that can be used indoors or outdoors. Adopt the boxer's style with both feet leaving the deck simultaneously. Marine women set a tempo of 80 to 100 jumps per minute. However, to jump continuously, set a pace that is realistic and appropriate to your current state of fitness. Gradually add 1 minute to your workout while increasing the tempo and intensity. If you prefer the rope jump but your ceiling is too low for indoor jumping, try simulating the action.

Cycling:

Bicycling, like running, pumps up the pulse, but you should not assume that a leisurely bike ride is productive. Although an easy ride may be advisable for anyone emerging from a sedentary lifestyle, cycling must be intense enough to produce a vigorous workout.

Generally, you can apply the same rules to cycling as you do to the walk/run. Begin with a cycling rhythm that warms you up and then increase your speed. If you feel comfortable, you are not working hard enough. If you get breathless, drop back to a slower place. When you have recovered, put in a little more effort again.

Stationary Cycling:

The stationary bicycle has proved to be effective in developing cardiorespiratory fitness, and, in fact, has some advantages over a mobile bicycle. The intensity of the workout on a stationary bicycle can be maintained, while a person riding the streets may be interrupted by traffic and be dependent on upgrades to increase the intensity. Also, it is easier to get on and off a stationary bicycle when rotating your cardiorespiratory workout with calisthenics in the 3X plan.

Adjust the height of the seat to get a full leg stroke. Pedal off the balls of your feet. This will help keep your feet straight. After a warmup of 3 to 5 minutes, increase the bike's resistance. If you have no problem keeping your balance, practice pumping your arms along your sides while simultaneously cycling. This raises your pulse further. When you feel secure moving your arms and legs at the same time, pump light dumbbells, 1 to 5 pounds.

Swimming:

Both the arms and legs are at work in the pool and this makes swimming an excellent cardiorespiratory conditioner. Swimming, however, can quickly fatigue the beginner, and the rule in cardiorespiratory conditioning is sustained workouts for 30 minutes and not less than 10 minutes. Therefore, the workout should be at a moderate but steady pace. Marines strongly recommend against swimming in the same time period with calisthenics, weight training and other land exercises. If you swim immediately after land conditioning, you may suffer cramps that are severe enough to cause drowning, and working out immediately after a swim may cause muscle and tissue damage. For these reasons, swimming should not be included in 3-cycle workouts.

Note: Swimming, cross-country skiing, long-distance running and bicycling are virtually the only weekend sports that provide satisfactory cardiorespiratory workouts. Look at it this way: cardiorespiratory conditioning will improve your sports performance, but most sports contribute little to cardiorespiratory efficiency.

PUTTING IT TOGETHER

ONCE you have compiled your starting levels, you can put together a 3-cycle conditioning format that the Corps has found to be effective in developing quality fitness for men and women.

The 3-cycle workout is also exceptionally efficient in gradually overloading the body because the procedure has a built-in safety factor: the intensity of the workout is regulated by your capacity, not the conditioning level of someone else.

In addition, the sequence of exercises is designed to work one group of muscles at a time. For example, while you exercise the lower torso, the upper torso is at rest.

The 3-Cycle Maximum-Effort Workout

The 3-Cycle Maximum-Effort Workout, popular with Marine men and women, is also used in training at the Officer Candidates School. It is a goal-oriented, no-frills workout based on a single, direct rule: in every cycle, you must make the effort to execute a maximum number of repetitions in each exercise.

The Max-Effort Workout

Cycle #1

1. Triceps Dips or Modified Dips: Maximum Performance
2. Pushups or Modified Pushups: Maximum Performance
3. Situps or Modified Situps: Maximum Performance
4. Pullups/Flexed-Arm Hangs or Modified Pullups/Hangs: Maximum Performance
5. Walk/Jog/Run: Maximum Performance

Cycle #2

Same as Cycle #1

Cycle #3

Same as Cycle #1

The 3-cycle format is a continuous workout with a rest break of 30 seconds or less between cycles. When you make a maximum effort in the first cycle, you are maintaining your current level of fitness. When you continue to make a maximum effort in the succeeding cycles, you are adding the overload necessary for progressive conditioning. Although you may not be able to execute as many repetitions or run as long in the second and third cycles, the sum of the 3 sets amounts to an overload that significantly increases strength and endurance. You can demonstrate this for yourself by recording your data on the chart below.

Personal Progress Chart for the Max-Effort Method

				Maximum Repetitions			
Date:	Level	Exercise	Goal	Cyc 1	Cyc 2	Cyc 3	Total
First Week:							
1. Triceps Dips or Modified Dips	___	___	___	___	___	___	___
2. Pushups or Modified Pushups	___	___	___	___	___	___	___
3. Situps or Modified Situps	___	___	___	___	___	___	___
4. Pullups/Flexed-Arm Hangs or Modified Pullups/Hangs*	___	___	___	___	___	___	___
5. Walk/Run Levels 1–3†	___	___	___	___	___	___	___

* Record Flexed-Arm Hangs in seconds.
† Record Walk/Run in minutes. See page 55 for chart to record higher levels of Walk/Run.

				Maximum Repetitions			
Date:	Level	Exercise	Goal	Cyc 1	Cyc 2	Cyc 3	Total
Fifth Week:							
1. Triceps Dips or Modified Dips	___	___	___	___	___	___	___
2. Pushups or Modified Pushups	___	___	___	___	___	___	___
3. Situps or Modified Situps	___	___	___	___	___	___	___
4. Pullups/Flexed-Arm Hangs or Modified Pullups/Hangs*	___	___	___	___	___	___	___
5. Walk/Run Levels 1–3†	___	___	___	___	___	___	___

* Record Flexed-Arm Hangs in seconds.
† Record Walk/Run in minutes. See page 55 for chart to record higher levels of Walk/Run.

Begin by testing and recording your maximum effort in each of the 3 cycles in each exercise listed in the chart. Then, at 4-, 5- or 6-week intervals, test again and record your progress.

The Maximum-Effort Workout has an additional advantage for anyone who hates paperwork. You can forget the chart. As long as you do your level best and go for the maximum, the overload will be continuous and the conditioning will be effective. When you execute the goal figure in any single cycle, move up to the next level of exercise.

For example, if you are working at Level 1 of upper-body conditioning, you will perform as many Off-the-Wall Pushoffs as possible in each cycle. As your strength and endurance improve, you will execute more pushoffs. When you reach your goal, 20 continuous repetitions in any single cycle, move up to Level 2.

Depending on your current condition, allow up to 30 seconds for recovery between each exercise and cycle. As your fitness improves, enabling you to work at a moderate to fast pace, walk/run-in-place for about 30 seconds during the recovery period, or move from one exercise to the next without pause. This helps to maintain your pulse at a workout level.

As noted earlier, Marines develop their own programs. You also have the option of modifying your cyclic workouts to your personal requirements.

Variations in 3-Cycle Workouts

An alternative to the 3-Cycle Max procedure, also recommended by the Officer Candidates School, is the 3-cycle Test-Retest Workout.

The 3-Cycle Test-Retest Workout

The Test-Retest workout is a simple but ingenious format that assures a progressive, 50% overload for muscle conditioning, no matter what your present state of fitness may be. This is the 3-step procedure:

Step 1: Test and record your maximum performance in each exercise category and enter the results in the Max-Effort column in the chart on page 53.

Step 2: Divide each of the Max-Effort figures by 2 and enter the results in column titled 50% Max. These entries tell you how many repetitions to execute in each cycle. For example, if your best performance at Level 4 in lower-body conditioning is 14 sidearm situps, execute 7 in each of 3 cycles for a total of 21. That ensures progressive conditioning with a 50% overload.

Step 3: Every 4 to 5 weeks, or whenever you find yourself performing any single exercise in the 3-cycle workout with ease, return to Step 1. Retest for your new maximum performance and upgrade your workout according to the instructions in Step 2. When your maximum effort meets that level's goal, move on to the next level. For example, when you can execute 20 continuous sidearm situps, move up to Level 5, hip situps, and test for your maximum effort in performing hip situps following Steps 1 and 2.

The following example of a 3-cycle workout is based on 50% of the maximum effort of a person who executed:

4 repetitions of Off-the-Block Dips
12 repetitions of Wall Pushoffs
14 repetitions of Sidearm Situps
2 repetitions of Chest-High Pullups

The Test-Retest Workout

Warmup

Cycle #1:

1. Off-the-Block Dips (Level 2): 2 repetitions
2. Wall Pushoffs (Level 1): 6 repetitions
3. Sidearm Situps (Level 3): 7 repetitions
4. Chest-High Pullups (Level 1): 1 repetition
5. Walk/Jog (Level 3—Walk 50/Jog 50): 10 minutes of your best effort

Cycle #2

Same as Cycle #1

Cycle #3

Same as Cycle #1

Cooldown

Three cycles add up to 6 repetitions of off-the-block dips, 18 repetitions of wall pushoffs, 21 repetitions of sidearm situps, and 3 repetitions of chest-high pullups. That amounts to a 50% overload for each exercise and a safe, dynamic conditioning program.

Your program may be planned and recorded by preparing a chart as shown on page 53.

Whether you choose the Max or Test-Retest procedure may depend on your temperament, the way you organize activities and your present state of conditioning. You may decide to start off with the test-retest procedure and switch to the maximum-effort workout at the maintenance level. It doesn't matter. Both produce excellent results.

The 3-cycle workout may also be adapted to available exercise equipment. If you don't have the use of horizontal bars, substitute off-the-bench dips for triceps dips; eliminate pullups and flexed-arm hangs.

Warmup

Cycle #1
1. Off-the-Bench (or Sofa) Dips
2. Situps or Modified Situps

Personal Progress Chart for the Test-Retest Method

Date: First Week:	Level	Exercise	Goal	Max Effort	50% Max
1. Triceps Dips or Modified Dips	——	——	——	——	——
2. Pushups or Modified Pushups	——	——	——	——	——
3. Situps or Modified Situps	——	——	——	——	——
4. Pullups/Flexed-Arm Hangs or Modified Pullups/Hangs*	——	——	——	——	——
5. Walk/Run Levels 1–3†	——	——	——	——	(Not applicable)

* Record Flexed-Arm Hangs in seconds.
† Record Walk/Run in minutes. See page 55 for chart to record higher levels of Walk/Run.

Date: Fifth Week:	Level	Exercise	Goal	Max Effort	50% Max
1. Triceps Dips or Modified Dips	——	——	——	——	——
2. Pushups or Modified Pushups	——	——	——	——	——
3. Situps or Modified Situps	——	——	——	——	——
4. Pullups/Flexed-Arm Hangs or Modified Pullups/Hangs*	——	——	——	——	——
5. Walk/Run Levels 1–3†	——	——	——	——	(Not applicable)

* Record Flexed-Arm Hangs in seconds.
† Record Walk/Run in minutes. See page 55 for chart to record higher levels of Walk/Run.

Date: Ninth Week:	Level	Exercise	Goal	Max Effort	50% Max
1. Triceps Dips or Modified Dips	——	——	——	——	——
2. Pushups or Modified Pushups	——	——	——	——	——.
3. Situps or Modified Situps	——	——	——	——	——
4. Pullups/Flexed-Arm Hangs or Modified Pullups/Hangs*	——	——	——	——	——
5. Walk/Run Levels 1–3†	——	——	——	——	(Not applicable)

* Record Flexed-Arm Hangs in seconds.
† Record Walk/Run in minutes. See page 55 for chart to record higher levels of Walk/Run.

3. Pushups or Modified Pushups
4. Walk/Jog/Run: 10 minutes

Cycle #2

Same as above

Cycle #3

Same as above

Cooldown

In the 3-cycle workouts shown above, the 10-minute walk/run is at the end of each sequence. This allows the skeletal muscles a chance to recover before beginning the next cycle of calisthenics. However, as you move into higher levels of cardiorespiratory conditioning, the length of running time extends beyond 10 minutes. If you turn back to page 45 of the cardiorespiratory program, you find that your goal at Level 6 is running 1.5 miles in 15 to 18 minutes. Because two 15-minute workouts are sufficient for basic cardiorespiratory conditioning, you may eliminate the walk/run workout in the third set and finish with a cooldown using the variation below:

Advanced 3-Cycle Workouts

Warmup

Cycle #1
1. Triceps Dips or Modified Dips
2. Situps or Modified Situps
3. Pushups or Modified Pushups
4. Pullups/Flexed-Arm Hangs or Modified Pullups/Hangs
5. Walk/Jog/Run: 1.5 Miles

Cycle #2

Same as above

Cycle #3

Same as above, but omit Walk/Jog/Run and execute Cooldown

The following chart will serve to record your cardiorespiratory progression for levels 4 through 9, when running is measured in both time and distance.

Cardiorespiratory Progress Chart

		Date	Distance In Miles	Actual Time In Minutes	Goal
Level 4	Run/Walk	____	1.0	_____	11
Level 5	Run/Walk	____	1.0	_____	10
Level 6	Run/Walk	____	1.5	_____	15–18
Level 7	Run/Walk	____	2.0	_____	20–23
Level 8	Run/Walk	____	2.5	_____	24–27
Level 9	Run/Walk	____	3.0	_____	28–30

When you enter Level 7 of cardiorespiratory conditioning, and begin to run 20 or more minutes, you have 2 options:

OPTION #1

3-Cycle Advanced Workout

Warmup

1. Triceps Dips or Modified Dips
2. Situps or Modified Situps
3. Pushups or Modified Pushups
4. Pullups/Flexed-Arm Hangs or Modified Pullups/Hangs
   After completing 3 cycles of the above exercises, immediately move into the cardiorespiratory workout:
5. Walk/Run continuously for 30 minutes

Cooldown

Note that you may run-in-place or rest up to 30 seconds between skeletal exercises.

The second option is for anyone who prefers to schedule muscle and cardiorespiratory workouts at different times of the day:

OPTION #2

3-Cycle Advanced Workout

Warmup

1. Triceps Dips or Modified Dips
2. Situps or Modified Situps

3. Pushups or Modified Pushups
4. Pullups/Flexed-Arm Hangs or Modified Pullups/Hangs

Cooldown

Warmup

5. Walk/Run 30 or More Minutes

Cooldown

With the above option, you must schedule an additional warmup and cooldown as shown above.

WHAT YOU SHOULD KNOW AND DO ABOUT WARMING UP AND COOLING DOWN

THE warmup, a mixture of flexibility and stretch exercises, prevents shock to the body by preparing the cardiorespiratory system and skeletal muscles for a vigorous workout. The procedure limbers up the body, warming and stretching muscles, while gradually increasing the pulse.

The 5-Minute Warmup

Start off slowly, keeping in mind that warmups are not a challenge and do not require great intensity. Allow 1 minute for each of the 5 following exercises:

1. OFF-THE-WALL ACHILLES STRETCHER

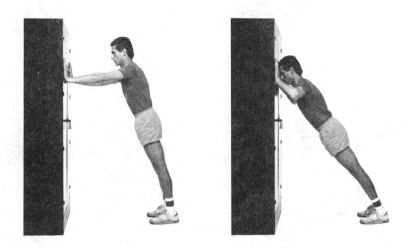

Purpose: To stretch the calf muscles, especially the large Achilles tendon, which runs from the heel bone to the calf muscle of the leg. This is useful as a warmup before running and is also an excellent stretch exercise for women who wear high heels. The Achilles Stretcher is useful in treating and preventing lower-limb injuries, including shin splints. The following exercise is a slight modification of the wall pushoff.

Starting Position: Stand a little more than arm's length from a wall with your feet toed in a little and slightly separated. Lean against the wall, supporting yourself with hands flat on the wall, palms pointed upward, arms straight. The key to effectiveness is keeping feet, including your heels, flat on the deck throughout the exercise.

Count 1:   Gradually bend your elbows outward. As you lean further into the wall you will feel your calf muscles stretch. Continue to ease forward until you feel these muscles pinching.

Count 2:   Hold this position for 5 to 10 seconds, then return to starting position.

Tempo: No cadence. Perform the exercise slowly, attending to the tension in your muscles. Repeat 10-second stretches for about a minute.

2. TOE TOUCHERS

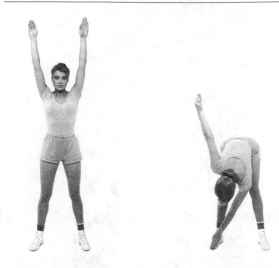

Purpose: To stretch the hamstrings, the muscles on the back of the thighs.
Starting Position: Upright with feet separated about shoulder-width. Arms over head.
Count 1: Touch toes of right foot with left hand.
Count 2: Return to starting position.
Count 3: Touch toes of left foot with right hand.
Count 4: Return to starting position.
Tempo: Begin easy, stretching slowly until muscles warm up. Continue alternating for a minute.

3. TRUNK TWIST

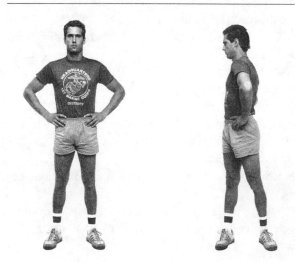

Purpose: Stretch obliques, hip extensors and upper legs.

Starting Position: Upright with feet comfortably separated. Hands on hips. Head up.

Count 1: Twist to left.

Count 2: Return to starting position.

Count 3: Twist to right.

Count 4: Return to starting position.

Tempo: Begin slowly, gradually stretching your muscles by twisting a little more on each count. Increase to moderate tempo and continue for a minute.

4. BEND AND REACH

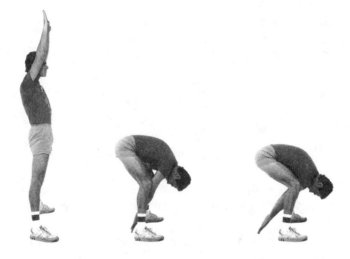

Purpose: To stretch the hip extensors and muscles of the upper leg.

Starting Position: Standing with feet comfortably separated—about the width of the hips for a woman, shoulder-width for a man. Arms are stretched above head with elbows locked and hands together.

Count 1: While bending at the knees, bring your arms down and reach backward between your knees and touch the deck.

Count 2: With a slight bounce, reach back as far as possible to touch the deck.

Count 3: Return to the starting position.

Tempo: Begin slowly, and gradually build up to a moderate pace. Continue for a minute.

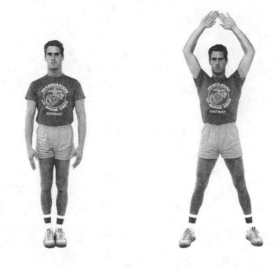

Purpose: To warm up the abductor and adductor muscles of the legs and shoulders, the muscles of the lower legs and ankles, and increase the pulse.
Starting Position: Standing, head up, with arms and hands along your sides.
Count 1: Jump off both feet, spreading your feet just slightly more than shoulder-width. At the same time swing your arms overhead until your hands touch.
Count 2: Jump again, swinging arms sideward and downward to your sides, returning to the starting position.
Tempo: Moderate to brisk. Continue for a minute.

The Cooldown

The cooldown is the easy part of an exercise period but important to your well-being. During a vigorous workout, blood concentrates in the muscles. If you stop exercising abruptly, you may feel dizzy, and perhaps faint, because the brain is short of blood. You may also have cramps and chills because lactic acid has accumulated in your muscles. These risks can be prevented with a simple cooling-off procedure.

If you are running hard, gradually reduce your speed from running to jogging and come down to a moderate walk until your pulse and breathing are normal. If you have been performing strength calisthenics, work the tension out of your muscles by rolling your shoulders, shaking your arms, stretching and bending. The cooldown should take about 5 minutes if you have been working hard, but you are the best judge of when your body is relaxed.

THE MAINTENANCE PHASE

PROGRESSIVE conditioning is virtually infinite. Fitness levels range from acceptable to shoot the moon. The mother of small children may require more endurance and agility than the woman executive. A weekend athlete requires a higher level of conditioning than the weekend spectator. College and professional athletes have to be in better shape than a weekend athlete, and an Olympic athlete shoots the moon.

Given many differences in lifestyles and goals, a maintenance program that sets the same fitness levels for everyone fails for most. For this reason, each person must decide according to his needs when to stop overloading and move into a maintenance program.

What Is Enough?

The goal of Marine conditioning is to bring men and women to a state of physical and mental readiness, which is defined as the ability to respond to the demands of the environment, whether it be a desk job or combat duty, single or family life. You can determine if your fitness matches Marine standards by taking the Physical Fitness Test in Part 3. You may also test yourself with the following questions:

· Are you alert on the job?
· Do you have the stamina for extra activities, such as sports or academic studies, dancing classes or hobbies, symposiums or social engagements, or merely to keep up with your family and home?
· Do you sleep well?
· Do you relax easily?

- Are you satisfied with your appearance, including your tone, posture and weight?
- Do you have the energy and strength to do your best throughout the day?
- Do you have the reserve to respond to a crisis or challenge with your best effort?
- Do you feel good about yourself?

You should be able to answer *yes* to these questions, because all of the benefits are reasonable and attainable goals. When you are feeling good about yourself and pass the fitness test, you may discontinue overloading whatever level you have reached. However, you must then go into a maintenance program, because the maxim "Use it or lose it" applies to physical fitness.

When workouts cease for 72 hours, deconditioning sets in and you lose the benefits listed above. To prevent this happening, all Marines follow a basic maintenance program.

The 3X Maintenance Formula

A basic program continues to maintain strength and endurance in three categories: upper torso, lower torso and cardiorespiratory. To accomplish this, Marines are required to schedule a minimum of three 60-minute workouts each week on alternate days.

The Corps recommends the following maintenance workout:

5 Minutes: The Warmup
15 Minutes: Strength and endurance exercises for skeletal muscles of the upper and lower body:
    a. Pullups/Chinups or Flexed-Arm Hangs
    b. Bent-Knee Situps
    c. Pushups
    d. Triceps Dips and/or Weight Training
35 Minutes: For cardiorespiratory efficiency, depending on individual capability, 3 to 5 miles of Run/Walk, or sprinting alternating with jogging.
5 Minutes: The Cooldown

(*Note:* Muscle and cardiorespiratory conditioning may be scheduled at different times of the day. If you choose this option, remember to include a warmup and a cooldown in both workouts.)

Your workout may also be a mix of progressive and maintenance conditioning. For example, you may be satisfied with conditioning in the lower body but dissatisfied with your upper body. In that case, settle on a fixed number of situp repetitions to maintain abdominal strength while continuing to overload your upper body with pushups, triceps dips and pullups.

You also have the option of competing with Marine standards. Officer candidates, who range in age from 20 to 29, schedule the following number of repetitions in 3-cycle workouts.

1. Situps	Men	3 sets of 40 repetitions
	Women	3 sets of 35 repetitions
2. Pushups	Men	3 sets of 30 repetitions
Pushups or Modified Pushups	Women	3 sets: maximum effort
3. Triceps Dips	Men	3 sets of 20 repetitions
	Women	3 sets of 10 repetitions
4. Pullups	Men	3 sets: maximum effort
Flexed-Arm Hangs	Women	3 sets: maximum effort
5. Run/Walk	Men	Up to 5 miles.
	Women	Up to 3 miles.

The above standards apply during the OCS training period. Once the candidate becomes an officer, fitness goals may differ. One Marine maintains fitness at an acceptable level, while another may shoot the moon. However, if you continue to perform the 3X cycle routinely and vigorously at an acceptable level, you have a program that will sustain your health and vigor for life. The formula is simple: 3 days a week, on alternate days, schedule a 3-cycle muscle and cardiorespiratory workout.

QUESTIONS AND ANSWERS

Q. Can I manipulate workouts for my convenience?

A. Yes. For example, you can exercise skeletal muscles on Monday, Wednesday and Friday, and schedule cardiorespiratory workouts on Tuesday, Thursday and Saturday. Also, the time of day does not matter. Because many Marines go on duty from 5 A.M. to 7 A.M., they usually schedule workouts during the lunch hour, late afternoon or early evening.

Q. How many hours should I allot?

A. During the preparatory and conditioning phases, the Corps states that 3 hours per week is mandatory and 5 hours, optimal. On a 3-hour-per-week program, schedule your 60-minute workouts on alternate days. Remember that each hour, whether in the conditioning or maintenance phase, must include a minimum of 30 to 35 minutes of cardiorespiratory conditioning. Of course, you achieve fitness goals more rapidly if you work out daily, although it is recommended that at least 1 day a week be put aside for rest.

Q. How will I know when I am not putting enough effort into a workout?

A. The comfort index is always your signal to exert more effort. If you feel comfortable, you are not working hard enough to condition your body. On the other hand, never hesitate to discontinue a workout if you feel pain. When beginners push to extremes, they become excessively fatigued, develop muscle soreness and headaches, and then become discouraged and quit.

Q. Can I substitute sports for the workout?

A. You cannot depend on a sport to maintain comprehensive fitness. Sports physiologists tell us, "You don't play games to get in shape. You get in shape to play." Conditioning improves your performance and prevents strains and sprains. However, using your fitness for recreation is strongly recommended. Marines use their conditioning to pursue personal activities, which may range from bodybuilding and boxing to tennis and aerobic dancing. If you engage in sports activities regularly, then schedule your games on days that alternate with your workouts: for example, Mondays, Wednesdays and Fridays for conditioning, and the alternate days for other physical activities.

Q. When should a maintenance program be reevaluated?

A. Once into the maintenance phase, you will come to enjoy a state of confidence that derives from good health and vigor. You should then be wary of activities requiring strength and endurance that go beyond your fitness level. For example, you may go on a vacation that includes rigorous physical activity, or you may jog with a friend who runs at a strenuous pace. Because you feel so good about yourself, you can overestimate your capacity. You won't get away with it. A sudden, sharp increase in physical activity can result in punishing pain or injury.

You can avoid a "jock's hangover" by anticipating the physical demands of an upcoming vacation or a seasonal sport. Prepare yourself by gradually increasing the overload during your workouts. Use the same procedure if your career requires longer, harder work hours, or if you decide to upgrade your weekend game.

The physical fitness tests that follow in Part 3 can be your guide in upgrading your conditioning. Begin by scoring your current fitness, and then retest yourself periodically to measure your progress.

· 3 ·

The Marine Physical Fitness Test

(INCLUDING YOUR SCORECARD)

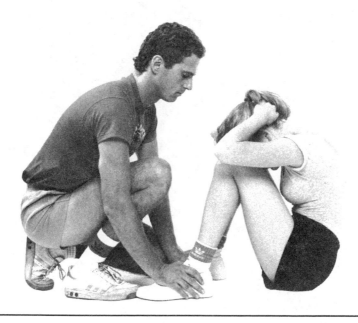

GO FOR IT!

MARINE Corps Order 6100.3H ". . . requires that every Marine, regardless of age, grade, or duty assignment, engage in an effective physical conditioning program on a continuing and progressive basis."

Why?

The regulation explains, "A program of regular, vigorous and progressive physical fitness training results in an increase in work efficiency, self-confidence, and personal as well as unit pride."

The regulation is specific about Marine objectives.

1. **Physical Fitness** is defined as a healthy body that can remain effective in prolonged activity even when it is necessary to endure discomforts and environmental stress for lengthy periods.

2. Therefore, **Stamina,** a combination of muscular and cardiorespiratory endurance, is considered the most important element in Marine fitness.

3. **Strength,** necessary for posture, work and confidence, is defined as the ability of an individual to manipulate her or his body weight.

What is most remarkable is that the Corps has developed a simple fitness test to determine if men and women meet the above goals. The test is generally administered semiannually, although a Marine must maintain the ability to pass the test at all times.

The Remarkable Test

For over a decade the Marine Physical Fitness Test has proved to be reliable, and this has been verified by independent research institutions. The Marine fitness test is also remarkable because it contains only 3 events:

3-Event Fitness Test

Category	Men	Women
Upper Torso:	Pullups	Flexed-Arm Hang
Lower Torso:	Situps	Situps
Cardiorespiratory and Legs:	3-Mile Run	1.5-Mile Run

The above events were chosen after study at the Research Laboratory of the Marine Corps Physical Fitness Laboratory. The object was to produce efficient field tests that would not require professional oversight. Many different events were considered.

The rope climb was eliminated as an upper-torso test because the evaluation of strength and endurance should not depend on an activity that is a learned skill. And because tests must have high reliability, the pullup and flexed-arm hang were chosen instead of the pushup, which is more likely to vary in execution from person to person.

The situp was chosen over the straight-leg lift, which does not bring as many abdominal muscles into full play. Runs have been designed to be long enough to test muscular endurance but short enough to predict cardiorespiratory fitness. Tests and scoring have been adjusted by age and sex, with minimum standards established for each group as illustrated in the following tables.

For Men Only: From Acceptable to Shoot the Moon

The Corps has set minimum standards for men by age group. In each event, the man must execute the minimum number of repetitions for each exercise and make the run in the minimum number of minutes. In addition, he must acquire enough additional points to earn a passing score.

Required Minimum Acceptable Performance for Men

Age	Pullups (no time limit)	Situps (2-minute limit)	3-Mile Run (in minutes)	Subtotal Points	Required Additional Points	Passing Score
17–26	3	40	28	95	40	135
27–39	3	35	29	84	26	110
40–45	3	35	30	78	7	85

If a man performs only the minimum in the 3 events, his subtotal, as illustrated in the above table, will fall short of the passing score. He must pick up additional points by exceeding the minimum performance in 1 or more of the 3 events. Note in the table below that the grand total also determines his class of fitness.

Required Minimum Scores for Men

Age	Unsatisfactory	3rd Class	2nd Class	1st Class
17–26	0–134	135	175	225
27–39	0–109	110	150	200
40–45	0–84	85	125	175

MAKING POINTS FOR FITNESS

The official Marine Scoring Table below applies to men in all age groups. The maximum score that can be achieved in any single event is 100 points; the maximum total score that can be achieved for all three events is 300 points.

Men's Scoring Table*

Points	Pullups	Situps	3-Mile Run	Points	Pullups	Situps	3-Mile Run	Points	Pullups	Situps	3-Mile Run	Points	Pullups	Situps	3-Mile Run
100	20	80	18:00	75	15		22:10	50	10	50	26:20	25	5	25	30:30
99			18:10	74		67	22:20	49		49	26:30	24		24	30:40
98		79	18:20	73			22:30	48		48	26:40	23		23	30:50
97			18:30	72		66	22:40	47		47	26:50	22		22	31:00
96		78	18:40	71			22:50	46		46	27:00	21		21	31:10
95	19		18:50	70	14	65	23:00	45	9	45	27:10	20	4	20	31:20
94		77	19:00	69			23:10	44		44	27:20	19		19	31:30
93			19:10	68		64	23:20	43		43	27:30	18		18	31:40
92		76	19:20	67			23:30	42		42	27:40	17		17	31:50
91			19:30	66		63	23:40	41		41	27:50	16		16	32:00
90	18	75	19:40	65	13		23:50	40	8	40	28:00	15	3	15	32:10
89			19:50	64		62	24:00	39		39	28:10	14		14	32:20
88		74	20:00	63			24:10	38		38	28:20	13		13	32:30
87			20:10	62		61	24:20	37		37	28:30	12		12	32:40
86		73	20:20	61			24:30	36		36	28:40	11		11	32:50
85	17		20:30	60	12	60	24:40	35	7	35	28:50	10	2	10	33:00
84		72	20:40	59		59	24:50	34		34	29:00	9		9	33:10
83			20:50	58		58	25:00	33		33	29:10	8		8	33:20
82		71	21:00	57		57	25:10	32		32	29:20	7		7	33:30
81			21:10	56		56	25:20	31		31	29:30	6		6	33:40
80	16	70	21:20	55	11	55	25:30	30	6	30	29:40	5	1	5	33:50
79			21:30	54		54	25:40	29		29	29:50	4		4	34:00
78		69	21:40	53		53	25:50	28		28	30:00	3		3	34:30
77			21:50	52		52	26:00	27		27	30:10	2		2	35:00
76		68	22:00	51		51	26:10	26		26	30:20	1		1	36:00

* All times that fall between the increments will receive the point value of the next longest time increment: for example, a time of 18:11 receives 98 points.

This is an example of how you go about scoring the men's events:

$$
\begin{aligned}
\text{4 pullups} &= \text{20 points} \\
\text{30 situps} &= \text{30 points} \\
\underline{\text{26:20 run}} &= \underline{\text{50 points}} \\
\text{Total Score:} &\quad \text{100 points}
\end{aligned}
$$

For Women Only: Minimal to Classy Fitness Standards

Marines have set minimum standards for women in each test event. Failing to meet the minimum requirement in a single event fails the whole test.

Required Minimum Acceptable Performance for Women

Age	Flexed- Arm Hang (in seconds)	Situps (1-minute limit) (Repetitions)	1.5-Mile Run (in minutes)	Earned Score
17–26	16	22	15	100
25–31	14	20	16	82
32–38	12	18	17	64
39–45	10	18	18	56

If a woman's performance is the bare minimum in each event, her earned score is acceptable and identifies her fitness category as 3rd class. When she can execute additional situps and better her time in the other events, her score increases, raising her fitness to classier levels.

Required Minimum Scores for Women

Age	Unsatisfactory	3rd Class	2nd Class	1st Class
17–24	0–99	100	150	200
25–31	0–81	82	132	182
32–38	0–63	64	114	164
39–45	0–55	56	106	156

MAKING POINTS FOR FITNESS

The official Marine Scoring Table below applies to women in all age groups. The maximum score that can be achieved in any single event is 100 points; the maximum that can be achieved for all three events is 300 points.

Points	Flexed-Arm Hang	Situps	1.5-Mile Run	Points	Flexed-Arm Hang	Situps	1.5-Mile Run	Points	Flexed-Arm Hang	Situps	1.5-Mile Run	Points	Flexed-Arm Hang	Situps	1.5-Mile Run
100	70	50	10:00	75			12:05	50	45	25	14:10	25	25		16:15
99			:05	74	57	37	:10	49			:15	24	24	12	:20
98	69	49	:10	73			:15	48	44	24	:20	23	23		:25
97			:15	72	56	36	:20	47			:25	22	22	11	:30
96	68	48	:20	71			:25	46	43	23	:30	21	21		:35
95			:25	70	55	35	:30	45			:35	20	20	10	:40
94	67	47	:30	69			:35	44	42	22	:40	19	19		:45
93			:35	68	54	34	:40	43			:45	18	18	9	:50
92	66	46	:40	67			:45	42	41	21	:50	17	17		16:55
91			:45	66	53	33	:50	41			14:55	16	16	8	17:00
90	65	45	:50	65			12:55	40	40	20	15:00	15	15		:10
89			10:55	64	52	32	13:00	39	39		:05	14	14	7	:20
88	64	44	11:00	63			:05	38	38	19	:10	13	13		:30
87			:05	62	51	31	:10	37	37		:15	12	12	6	:40
86	63	43	:10	61			:15	36	36	18	:20	11	11		17:50
85			:15	60	50	30	:20	35	35		:25	10	10	5	18:00
84	62	42	:20	59			:25	34	34	17	:30	9	9		:10
83			:25	58	49	29	:30	33	33		:35	8	8	4	:20
82	61	41	:30	57			:35	32	32	16	:40	7	7		:30
81			:35	56	48	28	:40	31	31		:45	6	6	3	:40
80	60	40	:40	55			:45	30	30	15	:50	5	5		18:50
79			:45	54	47	27	:50	29	29		15:55	4	4	2	19:00
78	59	39	:50	53			13:55	28	28	14	16:00	3	3	1	:30
77			11:55	52	46	26	14:00	27	27		:05	2	2	1	20:00
76	58	38	12:00	51			:05	26	26	13	:10	1	1		:30

* All times that fall between the increments will receive the point value of the next longest time increment: for example, a time of 10:11 receives 97 points.

This is an example of how you go about scoring the women's events:

30 seconds, flexed-arm hang	=	30 points
30 situps	=	60 points
15:15 minutes, 1.5-mile run	=	37 points
Total Score:		127 points

The Test: Doing It Right

The Corps schedules the entire fitness test for a single session with an adequate rest permitted between events. The length of the rest period is not critical, because each event tests a different region of the body. The run is always last, but the other events may be scheduled in any order.

The test may be performed without assistance, if you wish. The only equipment required is a horizontal chinning bar with a diameter of 1 to 1¾ inches. The bar is placed at a height well above your reach. Use a box or stool to step up to the bar, or you may be assisted by a companion. You will also need a stopwatch or a digital timepiece with a stopwatch function. Garments and shoes should be appropriate for exercising and running.

SITUPS: A TEST EVENT FOR BOTH MEN AND WOMEN

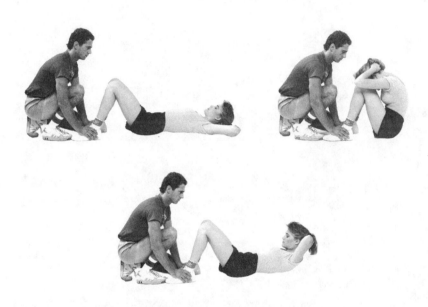

Time Limit: 1 minute for women; 2 minutes for men.

The Test: Lie flat on your back with fingers interlaced behind your head and touching the deck. Legs should be spread to about shoulder-width with knees bent. The correct angle of your thighs to the deck is about 45 degrees. Both feet must be flat on the deck, anchored under a barbell or sofa; during the actual Marine test, the person is held in place by an assistant. The assistant may hold the person's feet, grasp the legs below the knees or sit or kneel on the person's feet.

From the starting position, bend at the waist, raising the upper body from the supine position until your head breaks an imaginary plane through the knees. Heels must not leave the deck. To complete one repetition, lower your back until your shoulder blades touch the deck; neither your hands nor head need touch. Repeat the situp as many times as possible within the time limit.

Resting during the test in either the up or down position is permitted, but you cannot extend the specified time limit.

PULLUPS/CHINUPS: A TEST EVENT FOR MEN

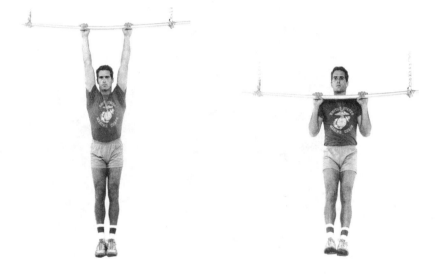

Time Limit: None.

The Test: The horizontal bar may be grasped with either an overhand or underhand grip but both palms must face the same direction. In the starting position, arms and legs are fully extended, with feet off the deck. One complete repetition requires using your arms to (1) pull up your body, raising your chin slightly over the bar, and (2) lower your body to the starting position. Repeat as many times as possible.

Because the horizontal bar will be out of your reach, you may be assisted into the hanging position by a companion, or use a box or stool to step up. If you jump to reach the bar, you may not use the momentum to perform your first pullup. Each pullup must start from the "dead man" hanging position. You may use kicking motions that do not raise above the waist. You can grunt and curse to your heart's content but you cannot swing your body when chinning.

You may change the position of your hands during the test if it can be done without dismounting or assistance. You may rest in either the down or up position, but you cannot use your chin for support or touch your feet to the deck, box or any other object.

The test ends when you drop to the deck.

FLEXED-ARM HANG: A TEST EVENT
FOR WOMEN

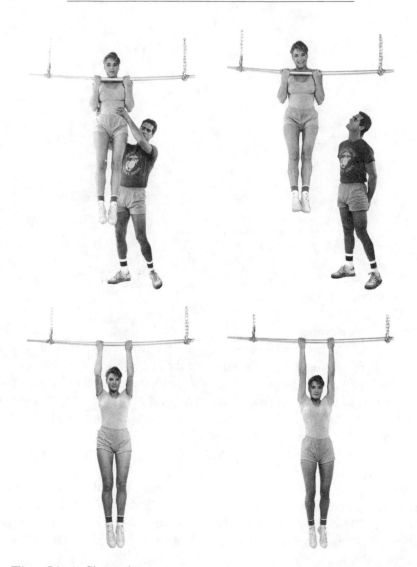

Time Limit: Shoot the moon.

The Test: The flexed-arm hang starts with your chin over or level with the horizontal bar but not touching the bar. You may have an assistant boost you into the flexed-arm position, or use either a box or stool to step up to the bar. Your feet must hang free.

The test is based on the number of seconds that you can maintain elbow flexion. Do not start the clock until the support is removed. When your arms are straight, the clock stops. You may use either the overhand or underhand grip, but both palms must face the same direction. During the test your chin may not rest on the bar.

THE RUN: A TEST EVENT FOR
MEN AND WOMEN

For women, a 1.5-mile measured course; for men, a 3-mile course. If a measured course is not available in a gym or park, use an automobile odometer to measure off the distance. Note that you may be better off circling the same block than running traffic lights.

The goal is to run the course in as little time as possible. You can easily compute your time in minutes and seconds with either a stopwatch or digital sports watch.

You may alternate walking with running if you wish. See page 41 for information on running form.

The PFT Scorecard

The Marine conditioning program is foolproof. You can confirm this by recording your progress. Begin by using the Marine Physical Fitness Test to determine your present level of conditioning, record the results, and then schedule retests at 6-week intervals. When you reach the maintenance level, mark a calendar to remind you to schedule tests quarterly or semiannually.

Record your progress in the chart below, a replica of a form commonly used by Marines, modified to include body-composition data:

Physical Fitness Test Scorecard

Fitness Events	Date _____ Performance	Score	Date _____ Performance	Score
Pullups/Flexed-Arm Hang:	_____	____	_____	____
Situps:	_____	____	_____	____
Run/Walk:	_____	____	_____	____
	Total Score:	____	Total Score:	____

Body Composition

Date _____ Date _____

Total Body Weight: _____ Total Body Weight: _____

% Body Fat: _____ % Body Fat: _____

	Date _____		Date _____	
	Performance	Score	Performance	Score
Fitness Events				
Pullups/Flexed-Arm Hang:	_____	_____	_____	_____
Situps:	_____	_____	_____	_____
Run/Walk:	_____	_____	_____	_____
	Total Score:	_____	Total Score:	_____

Body Composition

Date _____ Date _____

Total Body Weight: _____ Total Body Weight: _____

% Body Fat: _____ % Body Fat: _____

The fitness scoreboard calls for data on body composition because the percentage of body fat in your body is directly related to stamina, strength and appearance. An accurate method of assessing body composition follows in Part 4.

· 4 ·

The Marine Body-Fat Test

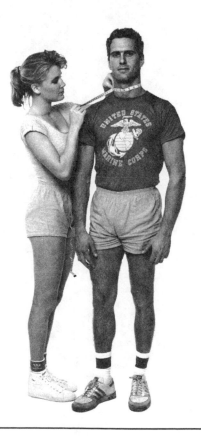

TO IMPROVE APPEARANCE, HEALTH, AND PERFORMANCE

No other institution takes the problem of body fat more seriously than the Marine Corps. An overweight Marine receives a grace period to lose excess fat. If there is no loss, regulations require that the Marine be discharged regardless of age, sex, grade or rank.

The Corps insists on a lean physique for the following reasons:

· To reduce the risk of incurring major health problems.
· To dramatically improve function, including agility, efficiency, strength and endurance.
· To maintain the Marines' traditional pride in appearance.

The Corps concern with overweight problems led to the development of a simple but accurate method of analyzing body composition. The technique, used to assess a person's percentage of body fat, is far more helpful in dealing with weight problems than the height-weight tables found on public scales and commonly used by insurance companies, health therapists and most military services.

A height-weight table lists only total body weight, or scale weight. Scale weight, however, does not tell you the percentage of body weight that is fat and the percentage that is lean mass, such as muscles, bones and other fat-free body parts. As a result, weight charts may be misleading. A study of nearly 300 Marines, age 18 to 53, from the grade of private to the rank of general, found that wrong conclusions may be drawn from height-weight tables. This is illustrated by data on 2 Marines who had the same weight and height but different body composition:

	First Marine	Second Marine
Height	73 inches	73 inches
Total Body Weight	227 pounds	227 pounds

According to height-weight tables (see page 94) both Marines should lose 18 pounds, but an analysis of their body composition finds a major difference between the 2 men.

	First Marine	*Second Marine*
Lean Body Weight	193.2 pounds	168.4 pounds
Fat Body Weight	33.8 pounds	58.6 pounds
Percent Body Fat	14.9%	25.8%

Although both have the same total weight, the first Marine has significantly less body fat and more lean body mass. Furthermore, his percentage of body fat, 14.9, falls well within acceptable allowances. The second Marine's percentage of body fat is excessive and will interfere with performance.

Civilian studies have found similar misleading conclusions based on height-weight tables. For example, a study of professional football players showed that the majority were classified as being grossly overweight according to height-weight tables. However, an analysis of their body composition found that these athletes were high in lean body mass, low in body fat and, furthermore, carried a smaller percentage of body fat than the average male college student.

To conform to the recommendations of height-weight tables, most of the professional athletes would have been forced to lose 20 to 40 pounds of lean mass. That would have been a mistake because we know that body fat, not lean mass, is the villain in health and performance.

For all of us, the question is: how much of our body fat is dead weight?

What Body Fat is Good For and When It's Nothing but Trouble

Both men and women are considered grossly obese when 30% or more of their total weight is fat; 20 to 30% body fat is likely to interfere with function, especially for a Marine and anyone else who is physically active. We have always known that obese people are likely to be sluggish. In recent years, we have also learned that a lean physique is a requisite for anyone who excels in physical activities.

The professional football study found that players' body fat ranges in the low 8% to 10% for backs and wide receivers, and from 10% to 16% for linemen. Some marathon runners are reported to carry under 8% and as little as 2% body fat. Research of women athletes finds that college swimmers average 13% to 19% body fat, and gymnasts average 11% to 15% body fat, although Olympic competitors have far less. Furthermore, studies find that the reduction of body fat by only 1% or 2% in already lean athletes often increases their power: the athletes swim, skate and run faster, kick and hit a ball farther and throw a ball harder.

Because a great body of research proves that performance, health and appearance are directly related to the body's composition, the Marine Corps has established body-fat standards for men and women of all ages:

- *18% is the maximum allowable percentage of body fat for male Marines, although their actual average is lower.* A study of the body composition of male Marines, age 18 to 53, from private to general, found that the men average 83.5% lean mass. Body fat was 16.5%, 1.5% below the acceptable allowance.
- *26% is the maximum allowable percentage of body fat for women Marines, although their actual average is lower.* A study of the body composition of women Marines, age 18 to 47, from private to general, found that the women average 76.9% lean mass. Body fat was 23.1%, about 3% below the acceptable allowance. (Note that women's sex characteristics account for a higher percentage of acceptable body fat.)

Your Goal: Decreasing body fat to maximum allowance and perhaps lower. How much lower is a personal decision, because no one can dictate an exact figure. The decision should be based on satisfaction with your health, performance and feelings about yourself.

The Marine Body-Fat Test

To assess an individual's body fat, the Corps developed a field test based on anthropometry, which is the technique of measuring the external parts of the body such as the thickness of a skin fold or the girth (circumference) of the neck, arm, waist or leg. For example, if you pinch your waist to get an idea of how much fat you have accumulated, you are gathering crude anthropometric data.

The Marine method of estimating body fat is based solely on girth measurements, a simple tool that can be used to anyone's advantage. When compared to the height-weight charts, which are considered primitive and inadequate by most experts, the anthropometric technique gives you a sophisticated assessment of your body's composition. All that you need is a tape measure and the tables that follow.

The Anthropometric Table for Men

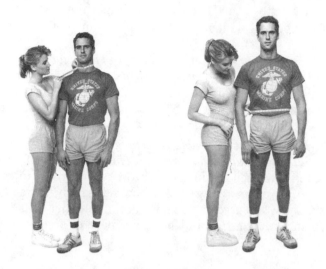

Two girth measurements are made to find a man's percentage of body fat, one at the waist and the other at the neck. When measuring, the tape should be taut and snug but not cut into the skin.

Neck: The neck circumference is measured just below the larynx (the Adam's apple) to the nearest quarter inch.

Waist: The waist circumference is measured at the navel to the nearest half inch. During the measurement, the man stands evenly on both legs while the stomach is held in a normal, relaxed position—*not* sucked in.

Match the waist measurement to the figures on the left side of the chart and the neck measurement to the figures at the top. Draw a line down from the neck measurement and a line across the chart from the waist measurement. Where the lines intersect, you find the assessment of a man's body fat. As an example:

Neck = 16 inches
Waist = 35 inches
BODY FAT = 15.6%

Percent Fat in Men from Waist and Neck Circumference

Neck (In.)

Abdomen (In.)	13.00	13.25	13.50	13.75	14.00	14.25	14.50	14.75	15.00	15.25	15.50	15.75	16.00	16.25
25.0	6.3	5.5	4.7	3.9	3.1	2.3	1.5	.7						
25.5	7.2	6.4	5.6	4.8	4.0	3.3	2.5	1.7	.9	.1				
26.0	8.2	7.4	6.6	5.8	5.0	4.2	3.4	2.6	1.8	1.0	.2			
26.5	9.1	8.3	7.5	6.7	5.9	5.1	4.3	3.5	2.8	2.0	1.2	.4		
27.0	10.0	9.2	8.4	7.7	6.9	6.1	5.3	4.5	3.7	2.9	2.1	1.3	.5	
27.5	11.0	10.2	9.4	8.6	7.8	7.0	6.2	5.4	4.6	3.8	3.0	2.3	1.5	.7
28.0	11.9	11.1	10.3	9.5	8.7	7.9	7.2	6.4	5.6	4.8	4.0	3.2	2.4	1.6
28.5	12.9	12.1	11.3	10.5	9.7	8.9	8.1	7.3	6.5	5.7	4.9	4.1	3.3	2.5
29.0	13.8	13.0	12.2	11.4	10.6	9.8	9.0	8.2	7.4	6.7	5.8	5.1	4.3	3.5
29.5	14.7	13.9	13.1	12.4	11.6	10.8	10.0	9.2	8.4	7.6	6.8	6.0	5.2	4.4
30.0	15.7	14.9	14.1	13.3	12.5	11.7	10.9	10.1	9.3	8.5	7.7	6.9	6.2	5.4
30.5	16.6	15.8	15.0	14.2	13.4	12.6	11.8	11.1	10.3	9.5	8.7	7.9	7.1	6.3
31.0	17.6	16.8	16.0	15.2	14.4	13.6	12.8	12.0	11.2	10.4	9.6	8.8	8.0	7.2
31.5	18.5	17.7	16.9	16.1	15.3	14.5	13.7	12.9	12.1	11.4	10.6	9.8	9.0	8.2
32.0	19.4	18.6	17.8	17.1	16.3	15.4	14.7	13.9	13.1	12.3	11.5	10.7	9.9	9.1
32.5	20.4	19.6	18.8	18.0	17.2	16.4	15.6	14.8	14.0	13.2	12.4	11.6	10.9	10.1
33.0	21.3	20.5	19.7	18.9	18.1	17.3	16.6	15.8	15.0	14.2	13.4	12.6	11.8	11.0
33.5	22.3	21.5	20.7	19.9	19.1	18.3	17.5	16.7	15.9	15.1	14.3	13.5	12.7	11.9
34.0	23.2	22.4	21.6	20.8	20.0	19.2	18.4	17.6	16.8	16.1	15.3	14.5	13.7	12.9
34.5	24.1	23.4	22.5	21.8	21.0	20.2	19.4	18.6	17.8	17.0	16.2	15.4	14.6	13.8
35.0	25.1	24.3	23.5	22.7	21.9	21.1	20.3	19.5	18.7	17.9	17.1	16.3	15.6	14.8
35.5	26.0	25.2	24.4	23.6	22.8	22.0	21.3	20.5	19.7	18.9	18.1	17.3	16.5	15.7
36.0	27.0	26.2	25.4	24.6	23.8	23.0	22.2	21.4	20.6	19.8	19.0	18.2	17.4	16.6
36.5	27.9	27.1	26.3	25.5	24.7	23.9	23.1	22.3	21.5	20.8	20.0	19.2	18.4	17.6
37.0	28.8	28.0	27.2	26.5	25.7	24.9	24.1	23.3	22.5	21.7	20.9	20.1	19.3	18.5
37.5	29.8	29.0	28.2	27.4	26.6	25.8	25.0	24.2	23.4	22.6	21.8	21.0	20.3	19.5
38.0	30.7	29.9	29.1	28.3	27.5	26.7	26.0	25.2	24.4	23.6	22.8	22.0	21.2	20.4
38.5	31.7	30.9	30.1	29.3	28.5	27.7	26.9	26.1	25.3	24.5	23.7	22.9	22.1	21.3
39.0	32.6	31.8	31.0	30.2	29.4	28.6	27.8	27.0	26.2	25.5	24.7	23.8	23.1	22.3
39.5	33.5	32.7	31.9	31.2	30.4	29.6	28.8	28.0	27.2	26.4	25.6	24.8	24.0	23.2
40.0	34.5	33.7	32.9	32.1	31.3	30.5	29.7	28.9	28.1	27.4	26.5	25.7	25.0	24.2
40.5	35.4	34.6	33.8	33.0	32.2	31.4	30.7	29.9	29.0	28.3	27.5	26.7	25.9	25.1
41.0	36.3	35.5	34.8	34.0	33.2	32.4	31.6	30.8	30.0	29.2	28.4	27.6	26.8	26.0
41.5	37.3	36.5	35.7	34.9	34.1	33.3	32.5	31.7	30.9	30.2	29.4	28.5	27.8	27.0
42.0	38.2	37.4	36.6	35.8	35.1	34.2	33.5	32.7	31.9	31.1	30.3	29.5	28.7	27.9
42.5	39.2	38.4	37.6	36.8	36.0	35.2	34.4	33.6	32.8	32.0	31.2	30.4	29.7	28.9
43.0	40.1	39.3	38.5	37.7	36.9	36.1	35.4	34.6	33.8	33.0	32.2	31.4	30.6	29.8
43.5	41.0	40.3	39.5	38.7	37.9	37.1	36.3	35.5	34.7	33.9	33.1	32.3	31.5	30.7
44.0	42.0	41.2	40.4	39.6	38.8	38.0	37.2	36.4	35.6	34.9	34.1	33.3	32.5	31.7
44.5	42.9	42.1	41.3	40.5	39.8	39.0	38.2	37.4	36.6	35.8	35.0	34.2	33.4	32.6
45.0	43.9	43.1	42.3	41.5	40.7	39.9	39.1	38.3	37.5	36.7	35.9	35.1	34.4	33.6
45.5	44.8	44.0	43.2	42.4	41.6	40.8	40.0	39.3	38.5	37.7	36.9	36.1	35.3	34.5
46.0	45.7	45.0	44.2	43.4	42.6	41.8	41.0	40.2	39.4	38.6	37.8	37.0	36.2	35.4
46.5	46.7	45.9	45.1	44.3	43.5	42.7	41.9	41.1	40.4	39.5	38.8	38.0	37.2	36.4
47.0	47.6	46.8	46.0	45.2	44.5	43.7	42.9	42.1	41.3	40.5	39.7	38.9	38.1	37.3
47.5	48.6	47.8	47.0	46.2	45.4	44.6	43.8	43.0	42.2	41.4	40.6	39.8	39.0	38.3
48.0	49.5	48.7	47.9	47.1	46.3	45.5	44.7	44.0	43.2	42.4	41.6	40.8	39.9	39.2
48.5	50.4	49.7	48.9	48.1	47.3	46.5	45.7	44.9	44.1	43.3	42.5	41.7	40.9	40.1
49.0	51.4	50.6	49.8	49.0	48.2	47.4	46.6	45.8	45.0	44.2	43.4	42.7	41.9	41.1
49.5	52.3	51.5	50.7	49.9	49.2	48.4	47.6	46.8	46.0	45.2	44.4	43.6	42.8	42.0
50.0	53.3	52.5	51.7	50.9	50.1	49.3	48.5	47.7	46.9	46.1	45.3	44.5	43.7	43.0

Percent Fat in Men from Waist and Neck Circumference

Neck (In.)

Abdomen (In.)	16.50	16.75	17.00	17.25	17.50	17.75	18.00	18.25	18.50	18.75	19.00	19.25	19.50	19.75
25.0														
25.5														
26.0														
26.5														
27.0														
27.5														
28.0	.8	.0												
28.5	1.8	1.0	.2											
29.0	2.7	1.9	1.1	.3										
29.5	3.6	2.8	2.0	1.3	.5									
30.0	4.6	3.8	3.0	2.2	1.4	.6								
30.5	5.5	4.7	3.9	3.1	2.3	1.5	.8							
31.0	6.5	5.6	4.9	4.1	3.3	2.5	1.7	.9	.1					
31.5	7.4	6.6	5.8	5.0	4.2	3.4	2.6	1.8	1.0	.3				
32.0	8.3	7.5	6.7	6.0	5.1	4.4	3.6	2.8	2.0	1.2	.4			
32.5	9.3	8.5	7.7	6.9	6.1	5.3	4.5	3.7	2.9	2.1	1.3	.5		
33.0	10.2	9.4	8.6	7.8	7.0	6.2	5.5	4.7	3.9	3.1	2.3	1.5	.7	
33.5	11.1	10.4	9.6	8.8	8.0	7.2	6.4	5.6	4.8	4.0	3.2	2.4	1.6	.8
34.0	12.1	11.3	10.5	9.7	8.9	8.1	7.3	6.5	5.7	5.0	4.2	3.4	2.6	1.8
34.5	13.0	12.2	11.4	10.6	9.9	9.1	8.3	7.5	6.7	5.9	5.1	4.3	3.5	2.7
35.0	14.0	13.2	12.4	11.6	10.8	10.0	9.2	8.4	7.6	6.8	6.0	5.2	4.5	3.7
35.5	14.9	14.1	13.3	12.5	11.7	10.9	10.1	9.4	8.6	7.8	7.0	6.2	5.4	4.6
36.0	15.8	15.1	14.3	13.5	12.7	11.9	11.1	10.3	9.5	8.7	7.9	7.1	6.3	5.5
36.5	16.8	16.0	15.2	14.4	13.6	12.8	12.0	11.2	10.4	9.6	8.9	8.1	7.3	6.5
37.0	17.7	16.9	16.1	15.3	14.6	13.8	13.0	12.2	11.4	10.6	9.8	9.0	8.2	7.4
37.5	18.7	17.9	17.1	16.3	15.5	14.7	13.9	13.1	12.3	11.5	10.7	9.9	9.2	8.4
38.0	19.6	18.8	18.0	17.2	16.4	15.6	14.8	14.1	13.3	12.5	11.7	10.9	10.1	9.3
38.5	20.5	19.8	19.0	18.2	17.4	16.6	15.8	15.0	14.2	13.4	12.6	11.8	11.0	10.2
39.0	21.5	20.7	19.9	19.1	18.3	17.5	16.7	15.9	15.1	14.3	13.6	12.8	12.0	11.2
39.5	22.4	21.6	20.8	20.0	19.3	18.5	17.7	16.9	16.1	15.3	14.5	13.7	12.9	12.1
40.0	23.4	22.6	21.8	21.0	20.2	19.4	18.6	17.8	17.0	16.2	15.4	14.6	13.8	13.1
40.5	24.3	23.5	22.7	21.9	21.1	20.3	19.5	18.7	18.0	17.2	16.4	15.6	14.8	14.0
41.0	25.2	24.5	23.7	22.9	22.1	21.3	20.5	19.7	18.9	18.1	17.3	16.5	15.7	14.9
41.5	26.2	25.4	24.6	23.8	23.0	22.2	21.4	20.6	19.8	19.0	18.2	17.4	16.7	15.9
42.0	27.1	26.3	25.5	24.7	24.0	23.2	22.3	21.5	20.8	20.0	19.2	18.4	17.6	16.8
42.5	28.1	27.3	26.5	25.7	24.9	24.1	23.3	22.5	21.7	20.9	20.1	19.3	18.5	17.8
43.0	29.0	28.2	27.4	26.6	25.8	25.0	24.2	23.4	22.7	21.9	21.1	20.3	19.5	18.7
43.5	29.9	29.2	28.4	27.6	26.8	26.0	25.2	24.4	23.6	22.8	22.0	21.2	20.4	19.6
44.0	30.9	30.1	29.3	28.5	27.7	26.9	26.1	25.3	24.5	23.7	23.0	22.2	21.4	20.6
44.5	31.8	31.0	30.2	29.4	28.7	27.9	27.1	26.3	25.5	24.7	23.9	23.1	22.3	21.5
45.0	32.8	32.0	31.2	30.4	29.6	28.8	28.0	27.2	26.4	25.6	24.8	24.0	23.2	22.5
45.5	33.7	32.9	32.1	31.3	30.5	29.7	28.9	28.2	27.4	26.6	25.8	25.0	24.2	23.4
46.0	34.6	33.9	33.1	32.3	31.5	30.7	29.9	29.1	28.3	27.5	26.7	25.9	25.1	24.3
46.5	35.6	34.8	34.0	33.2	32.4	31.6	30.8	30.0	29.2	28.4	27.7	26.9	26.1	25.3
47.0	36.5	35.7	34.9	34.1	33.4	32.6	31.8	31.0	30.2	29.4	28.6	27.8	27.0	26.2
47.5	37.5	36.7	35.9	35.1	34.3	33.5	32.7	31.9	31.1	30.3	29.5	28.7	27.9	27.2
48.0	38.4	37.6	36.8	36.0	35.2	34.4	33.6	32.9	32.1	31.3	30.5	29.7	28.9	28.1
48.5	39.3	38.5	37.8	37.0	36.2	35.4	34.6	33.8	33.0	32.2	31.4	30.6	29.8	29.0
49.0	40.3	39.5	38.7	37.9	37.1	36.3	35.5	34.7	33.9	33.1	32.4	31.6	30.8	30.0
49.5	41.2	40.4	39.6	38.8	38.1	37.3	36.5	35.7	34.9	34.1	33.3	32.5	31.7	30.9
50.0	42.2	41.4	40.6	39.8	39.0	38.2	37.4	36.6	35.8	35.0	34.2	33.4	32.6	31.9

The Anthropometric Table for Women

A woman must make five girth measurements to determine how much of her total body weight is fat. The figures matched to the left of each girth measurement represent fat points. When measuring, the tape should be taut and snug but not cut into the skin. Read measurements to the nearest eighth inch.

Thigh: In this measurement, the woman should be balanced evenly on both legs with her feet slightly apart. The tape is placed just below the gluteal fold.
Enter fat points: _____

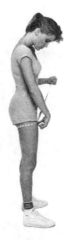

Biceps Extended: Measure the largest part of the bicep/triceps/muscle group with your arm held out from your body and your palm facing up. Note that the arm is straight and held at a 90-degree angle from the shoulder.
Enter fat points: _____

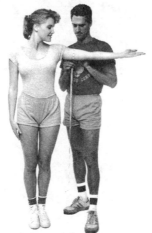

Thigh Measurement Table

Pts	*Thigh*	*Pts*	*Thigh*	*Pts*	*Thigh*	*Pts*	*Thigh*	*Pts*	*Thigh*
.0	11 6/8	7.0	16 2/8	13.7	20 6/8	20.5	25 2/8	27.3	29 6/8
.2	11 7/8	7.1	16 3/8	13.9	20 7/8	20.7	25 3/8	27.5	29 7/8
.4	12 0/8	7.3	16 4/8	14.1	21 0/8	20.9	25 4/8	27.7	30 0/8
.6	12 1/8	7.4	16 5/8	14.3	21 1/8	21.1	25 5/8	27.9	30 1/8
.8	12 2/8	7.6	16 6/8	14.5	21 2/8	21.3	25 6/8	28.1	30 2/8
1.0	12 3/8	7.8	16 7/8	14.6	21 3/8	21.5	25 7/8	28.3	30 3/8
1.2	12 4/8	8.0	17 0/8	14.8	21 4/8	21.7	26 0/8	28.5	30 4/8
1.4	12 5/8	8.2	17 1/8	15.0	21 5/8	21.8	26 1/8	28.7	30 5/8
1.6	12 6/8	8.4	17 2/8	15.2	21 6/8	22.0	26 2/8	28.9	30 6/8
1.8	12 7/8	8.6	17 3/8	15.4	21 7/8	22.2	26 3/8	29.0	30 7/8
1.9	13 0/8	8.8	17 4/8	15.6	22 0/8	22.4	26 4/8	29.2	31 0/8
2.1	13 1/8	9.0	17 5/8	15.8	22 1/8	22.6	26 5/8	29.4	31 1/8
2.3	13 2/8	9.1	17 6/8	16.0	22 2/8	22.8	26 6/8	29.6	31 2/8
2.5	13 3/8	9.3	17 7/8	16.2	22 3/8	23.0	26 7/8	29.8	31 3/8
2.7	13 4/8	9.5	18 0/8	16.3	22 4/8	23.2	27 0/8	30.0	31 4/8
2.9	13 5/8	9.7	18 1/8	16.5	22 5/8	23.4	27 1/8	30.2	31 5/8
3.1	13 6/8	9.9	18 2/8	16.7	22 6/8	23.6	27 2/8	30.4	31 6/8
3.3	13 7/8	10.1	18 3/8	16.9	22 7/8	23.7	27 3/8	30.6	31 7/8
3.5	14 0/8	10.3	18 4/8	17.1	23 0/8	23.9	27 4/8	30.8	32 0/8
3.6	14 1/8	10.5	18 5/8	17.3	23 1/8	24.1	27 5/8	30.9	32 1/8
3.8	14 2/8	10.7	18 6/8	17.5	23 2/8	24.3	27 6/8	31.1	32 2/8
4.0	14 3/8	10.9	18 7/8	17.7	23 3/8	24.5	27 7/8	31.3	32 3/8
4.2	14 4/8	11.0	19 0/8	17.9	23 4/8	24.7	28 0/8	31.5	32 4/8
4.4	14 5/8	11.2	19 1/8	18.1	23 5/8	24.9	28 1/8	31.7	32 5/8
4.6	14 6/8	11.4	19 2/8	18.2	23 6/8	25.1	28 2/8	31.9	32 6/8
4.8	14 7/8	11.6	19 3/8	18.4	23 7/8	25.3	28 3/8	32.1	32 7/8
5.0	15 0/8	11.8	19 4/8	18.6	24 0/8	25.4	28 4/8	32.3	33 0/8
5.2	15 1/8	12.0	19 5/8	18.8	24 1/8	25.6	28 5/8	32.5	33 1/8
5.4	15 2/8	12.2	19 6/8	19.0	24 2/8	25.8	28 6/8	32.7	33 2/8
5.5	15 3/8	12.4	19 7/8	19.2	24 3/8	26.0	28 7/8	32.8	33 3/8
5.7	15 4/8	12.6	20 0/8	19.4	24 4/8	26.2	29 0/8	32.9	33 4/8
5.9	15 5/8	12.7	20 1/8	19.6	24 5/8	26.4	29 1/8		
6.1	15 6/8	12.9	20 2/8	19.8	24 6/8	26.6	29 2/8		
6.3	15 7/8	13.1	20 3/8	20.0	24 7/8	26.8	29 3/8		
6.5	16 0/8	13.3	20 4/8	20.1	25 0/8	27.0	29 4/8		
6.7	16 1/8	13.5	20 5/8	20.3	25 1/8	27.2	29 5/8		

Biceps-Forearm Measurement Tables

Pts	*Biceps*	*Pts*	*Biceps*	*Pts*	*Biceps*	*Pts*	*Biceps*	*Pts*	*Biceps*
.1	5 7/8	4.8	7 5/8	9.4	9 3/8	14.1	11 1/8	18.8	12 7/8
.4	6 0/8	5.1	7 6/8	9.8	9 4/8	14.5	11 2/8	19.1	13 0/8
.8	6 1/8	5.4	7 7/8	10.1	9 5/8	14.8	11 3/8	19.5	13 1/8
1.1	6 2/8	5.8	8 0/8	10.4	9 6/8	15.1	11 4/8	19.8	13 2/8
1.4	6 3/8	6.1	8 1/8	10.8	9 7/8	15.5	11 5/8	20.1	13 3/8
1.8	6 4/8	6.4	8 2/8	11.1	10 0/8	15.8	11 6/8	20.5	13 4/8
2.1	6 5/8	6.8	8 3/8	11.4	10 1/8	16.1	11 7/8	20.8	13 5/8
2.4	6 6/8	7.1	8 4/8	11.8	10 2/8	16.5	12 0/8	21.1	13 6/8
2.8	6 7/8	7.4	8 5/8	12.1	10 3/8	16.8	12 1/8		
3.1	7 0/8	7.8	8 6/8	12.4	10 4/8	17.1	12 2/8		
3.4	7 1/8	8.1	8 7/8	12.8	10 5/8	17.5	12 3/8		
3.8	7 2/8	8.4	9 0/8	13.1	10 6/8	17.8	12 4/8		
4.1	7 3/8	8.8	9 1/8	13.5	10 7/8	18.1	12 5/8		
4.4	7 4/8	9.1	9 2/8	13.8	11 0/8	18.5	12 6/8		

Pts	*Forearm*	*Pts*	*Forearm*	*Pts*	*Forearm*	*Pts*	*Forearm*	*Pts*	*Forearm*
.2	17 5/8	9.3	15 2/8	18.5	12 7/8	27.7	10 4/8	36.8	8 1/8
.6	17 4/8	9.8	15 1/8	19.0	12 6/8	28.1	10 3/8	37.3	8 0/8
1.1	17 3/8	10.3	15 0/8	19.5	12 5/8	28.5	10 2/8	37.8	7 7/8
1.6	17 2/8	10.8	14 7/8	19.9	12 4/8	29.1	10 1/8	38.3	7 6/8
2.1	17 1/8	11.2	14 6/8	20.4	12 3/8	29.6	10 0/8	38.8	7 5/8
2.5	17 0/8	11.7	14 5/8	20.9	12 2/8	30.1	9 7/8	39.3	7 4/8
3.0	16 7/8	12.2	14 4/8	21.4	12 1/8	30.6	9 6/8	39.7	7 3/8
3.5	16 6/8	12.7	14 3/8	21.9	12 0/8	31.0	9 5/8	40.2	7 2/8
4.0	16 5/8	13.2	14 2/8	22.3	11 7/8	31.5	9 4/8	40.7	7 1/8
4.5	16 4/8	13.7	14 1/8	22.8	11 6/8	32.0	9 3/8	41.2	7 0/8
5.0	16 3/8	14.1	14 0/8	23.3	11 5/8	32.5	9 2/8	41.7	6 7/8
5.4	16 2/8	14.6	13 7/8	23.8	11 4/8	33.0	9 1/8	42.2	6 6/8
5.9	16 1/8	15.1	13 6/8	24.3	11 3/8	33.5	9 0/8	42.5	6 5/8
6.4	16 0/8	15.6	13 5/8	24.9	11 2/8	33.9	8 7/8	.0	0 0/8
6.9	15 7/8	16.1	13 4/8	25.2	11 1/8	34.4	8 6/8		
7.4	15 6/8	16.6	13 3/8	25.7	11 0/8	34.9	8 5/8		
7.9	15 5/8	17.0	13 2/8	26.2	10 7/8	35.4	8 4/8		
8.3	15 4/8	17.5	13 1/8	26.7	10 6/8	36.0	8 3/8		
8.8	15 3/8	18.0	13 0/8	27.2	10 5/8	36.4	8 2/8		

Forearm: Continue to hold your arm straight out from your shoulder with palm facing up, and measure the largest part of the forearm.
Enter fat points: _____

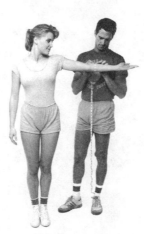

Neck: Measure the neck just below the larynx.
Enter fat points: _____

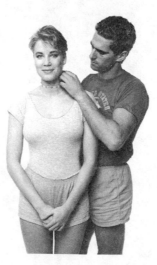

Neck Measurement Table

Pts	*Neck*	*Pts*	*Neck*	*Pts*	*Neck*	*Pts*	*Neck*	*Pts*	*Neck*
.1	15 5/8	4.1	13 7/8	8.0	12 1/8	11.9	10 3/8	15.8	8 5/8
.4	15 4/8	4.3	13 6/8	8.2	12 0/8	12.1	10 2/8	16.1	8 4/8
.7	15 3/8	4.6	13 5/8	8.5	11 7/8	12.4	10 1/8	16.3	8 3/8
1.0	15 2/8	4.9	13 4/8	8.8	11 6/8	12.7	10 0/8	16.7	8 2/8
1.3	15 1/8	5.2	13 3/8	9.1	11 5/8	13.0	9 7/8	16.9	8 1/8
1.5	15 0/8	5.4	13 2/8	9.4	11 4/8	13.3	9 6/8	17.2	8 0/8
1.8	14 7/8	5.7	13 1/8	9.6	11 3/8	13.5	9 5/8	17.4	7 7/8
2.1	14 6/8	6.0	13 0/8	9.9	11 2/8	13.8	9 4/8	17.7	7 6/8
2.4	14 5/8	6.3	12 7/8	10.2	11 1/8	14.1	9 3/8	18.0	7 5/8
2.7	14 4/8	6.6	12 6/8	10.6	11 0/8	14.4	9 2/8	18.3	7 4/8
2.9	14 3/8	6.8	12 5/8	10.8	10 7/8	14.7	9 1/8	18.6	7 3/8
3.2	14 2/8	7.1	12 4/8	11.0	10 6/8	14.9	9 0/8		
3.5	14 1/8	7.4	12 3/8	11.3	10 5/8	15.2	8 7/8		
3.8	14 0/8	7.7	12 2/8	11.6	10 4/8	15.5	8 6/8		

Abdomen: Measure at the level of the navel.
Enter fat points: ____

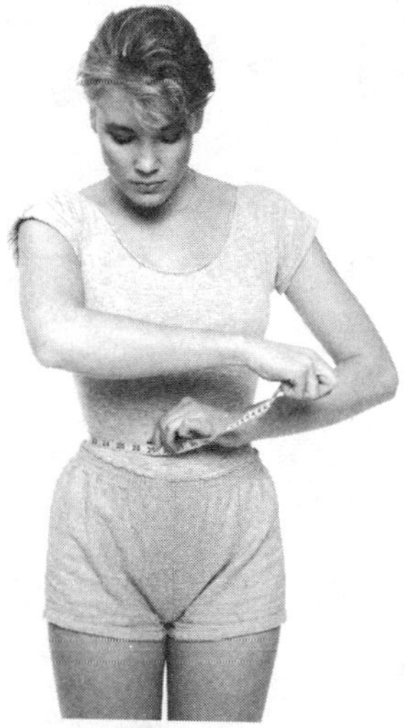

Add up the points accumulated from all five measurements. Subtract the constant correction factor 54.598 from the total. The resulting figure represents the percentage of fat in your body. This is an example:

	Inches	Points
Neck:	10 0/8 =	12.7
Abdomen:	28 0/8 =	8.6
Biceps:	12 4/8 =	17.8
Forearm:	11 0/8 =	25.7
Thigh:	19 0/8 =	11.0
	Total Points =	75.800
	Minus Correction Factor −	54.598
	BODY-FAT PERCENTAGE =	21.202

Abdomen Measurement Table

Pts	*Abdomen*	*Pts*	*Abdomen*	*Pts*	*Abdomen*	*Pts*	*Abdomen*	*Pts*	*Abdomen*	*Pts*	*Abdomen*
.0	17 5/8	4.4	23 0/8	8.9	28 3/8	13.3	33 6/8	17.8	39 1/8	22.2	44 4/8
.1	17 6/8	4.5	23 1/8	9.0	28 4/8	13.4	33 7/8	17.9	39 2/8	22.3	44 5/8
.2	17 7/8	4.6	23 2/8	9.1	28 5/8	13.5	34 0/8	18.0	39 3/8	22.4	44 6/8
.3	18 0/8	4.7	23 3/8	9.2	28 6/8	13.6	34 1/8	18.1	39 4/8	22.5	44 7/8
.4	18 1/8	4.8	23 4/8	9.3	28 7/8	13.7	34 2/8	18.2	39 5/8	22.6	45 0/8
.5	18 2/8	4.9	23 5/8	9.4	29 0/8	13.8	34 3/8	18.3	39 6/8	22.7	45 1/8
.6	18 3/8	5.0	23 6/8	9.5	29 1/8	14.0	34 4/8	18.4	39 7/8	22.9	45 2/8
.7	18 4/8	5.2	23 7/8	9.6	29 2/8	14.1	34 5/8	18.5	40 0/8	23.0	45 3/8
.8	18 5/8	5.3	24 0/8	9.7	29 3/8	14.2	34 6/8	18.6	40 1/8	23.1	45 4/8
.9	18 6/8	5.4	24 1/8	9.8	29 4/8	14.3	34 7/8	18.7	40 2/8	23.2	45 5/8
1.0	18 7/8	5.5	24 2/8	9.9	29 5/8	14.4	35 0/8	18.8	40 3/8	23.3	45 6/8
1.1	19 0/8	5.6	24 3/8	10.0	29 6/8	14.5	35 1/8	18.9	40 4/8	23.4	45 7/8
1.2	19 1/8	5.7	24 4/8	10.1	29 7/8	14.6	35 2/8	19.0	40 5/8	23.5	46 0/8
1.3	19 2/8	5.8	24 5/8	10.2	30 0/8	14.7	35 3/8	19.1	40 6/8	23.6	46 1/8
1.4	19 3/8	5.9	24 6/8	10.3	30 1/8	14.8	35 4/8	19.2	40 7/8	23.7	46 2/8
1.5	19 4/8	6.0	24 7/8	10.4	30 2/8	14.9	35 5/8	19.3	41 0/8	23.8	46 3/8
1.6	19 5/8	6.1	25 0/8	10.5	30 3/8	15.0	35 6/8	19.4	41 1/8	23.9	46 4/8
1.7	19 6/8	6.2	25 1/8	10.6	30 4/8	15.1	35 7/8	19.5	41 2/8	24.0	46 5/8
1.8	19 7/8	6.3	25 2/8	10.7	30 5/8	15.2	36 0/8	19.6	41 3/8	24.1	46 6/8
1.9	20 0/8	6.4	25 3/8	10.8	30 6/8	15.3	36 1/8	19.7	41 4/8	24.2	46 7/8
2.0	20 1/8	6.5	25 4/8	10.9	30 7/8	15.4	36 2/8	19.9	41 5/8	24.3	47 0/8

Pts	*Abdomen*	*Pts*	*Abdomen*	*Pts*	*Abdomen*	*Pts*	*Abdomen*	*Pts*	*Abdomen*	*Pts*	*Abdomen*
2.2	20⅖	6.6	25⅝	11.1	31⁰⁄₈	15.5	36⅜	20.0	41⁶⁄₈	24.4	47⅛
2.3	20⅜	6.7	25⁶⁄₈	11.2	31⅛	15.6	36⁴⁄₈	20.1	41⅞	24.5	47²⁄₈
2.4	20⁴⁄₈	6.8	25⅞	11.3	31²⁄₈	15.7	36⅝	20.2	42⁰⁄₈	24.6	47⅜
2.5	20⅝	6.9	26⁰⁄₈	11.4	31⅜	15.8	36⁶⁄₈	20.3	42⅛	24.7	47⁴⁄₈
2.6	20⁶⁄₈	7.0	26⅛	11.5	31⁴⁄₈	15.9	36⅞	20.4	42²⁄₈	24.8	47⅝
2.7	20⅞	7.1	26²⁄₈	11.6	31⅝	16.0	37⁰⁄₈	20.5	42⅜	24.9	47⁶⁄₈
2.8	21⁰⁄₈	7.2	26⅜	11.7	31⁶⁄₈	16.1	37⅛	20.6	42⁴⁄₈	25.0	47⅞
2.9	21⅛	7.3	26⁴⁄₈	11.8	31⅞	16.2	37²⁄₈	20.7	42⅝	25.1	48⁰⁄₈
3.0	21²⁄₈	7.4	26⅝	11.9	32⁰⁄₈	16.3	37⅜	20.8	42⁶⁄₈	25.2	48⅛
3.1	21⅜	7.5	26⁶⁄₈	12.0	32⅛	16.4	37⁴⁄₈	20.9	42⅞	25.3	48²⁄₈
3.2	21⁴⁄₈	7.6	26⅞	12.1	32²⁄₈	16.5	37⅝	21.0	43⁰⁄₈	25.4	48⅜
3.3	21⅝	7.7	27⁰⁄₈	12.2	32⅜	16.6	37⁶⁄₈	21.1	43⅛	25.5	48⁴⁄₈
3.4	21⁶⁄₈	7.8	27⅛	12.3	32⁴⁄₈	16.7	37⅞	21.2	43²⁄₈	25.6	48⅝
3.5	21⅞	7.9	27²⁄₈	12.4	32⅝	16.8	38⁰⁄₈	21.3	43⅜	25.8	48⁶⁄₈
3.6	22⁰⁄₈	8.1	27⅜	12.5	32⁶⁄₈	17.0	38⅛	21.4	43⁴⁄₈	25.9	48⅞
3.7	22⅛	8.2	27⁴⁄₈	12.6	32⅞	17.1	38²⁄₈	21.5	43⅝	26.0	49⁰⁄₈
3.8	22²⁄₈	8.3	27⅝	12.7	33⁰⁄₈	17.2	38⅜	21.6	43⁶⁄₈	26.1	49⅛
3.9	22⅜	8.4	27⁶⁄₈	12.8	33⅛	17.3	38⁴⁄₈	21.7	43⅞		
4.0	22⁴⁄₈	8.5	27⅞	12.9	33²⁄₈	17.4	38⅝	21.8	44⁰⁄₈		
4.1	22⅝	8.6	28⁰⁄₈	13.0	33⅜	17.5	38⁶⁄₈	21.9	44⅛		
4.2	22⁶⁄₈	8.7	28⅛	13.1	33⁴⁄₈	17.6	38⅞	22.0	44²⁄₈		
4.3	22⅞	8.8	28²⁄₈	13.2	33⅝	17.7	39⁰⁄₈	22.1	44⅜		

Weight-Standard Charts for Men and Women Regardless of Age

The following weight chart sets the standards for men:

Height (inches)	Weight (pounds) minimum	Weight (pounds) maximum
64	105	160
65	106	165
66	107	170
67	111	175
68	115	181
69	119	186
70	123	192
71	127	197
72	131	203
73	135	209
74	139	214
75	143	225
76	147	219
77	151	230
78	153	235

The following weight chart sets the standards for women:

Height (inches)	Weight (pounds) minimum	Weight (pounds) maximum
58	90	121
59	92	123
60	94	125
61	96	127
62	98	130
63	100	134
64	102	138
65	104	142
66	106	147
67	109	151
68	112	156
69	115	160
70	118	165
71	122	170
72	125	175
73	128	180

The above charts are used routinely by Marine commanders to identify anyone who exceeds the maximum allowable weight standards. However, if the "overweight" Marine performs satisfactorily, looks good and passes the physical fitness test, there is the probability that the person's body composition is low on body fat. The anthropometric method is then used to determine if the Marine's percentage of body fat falls within the acceptable limit.

QUESTIONS AND ANSWERS

Q. How important is a lean physique to a person's well-being?

A. A person's fitness, both mental and physical, is directly related to the percentage of fat in the body. Excess body fat affects the way that we feel about ourselves and the way others see us, which explains the Marine emphasis on appearance. The elimination of excess body fat is also a critical factor in improving our health and performance.

Q. When do you use the weight charts and when do you use the anthropometric method?

A. If, according to the weight chart, your scale weight is acceptable, and if you are healthy, energetic and can pass the physical fitness test, it's likely that your body-fat percentage falls into acceptable levels. However, the anthropometric data provides a more intelligent assessment of your body composition.

Actually, many of us already rely on anthropometric feedback. When our belts or the waistbands of our garments pinch, we know that we are putting on fat. With the Marine method, however, you not only assess your present percentage of body fat but you can also do some fine tuning, reducing body fat in small percentages until you reach your maximum performance.

Q. What's the danger in losing too much fat?

A. For most of us it is very difficult, if not genetically improbable, to get below 10% body fat. However, it is usually a good idea to check with your physician when beginning a weight-loss program, as Marines do, to eliminate the possibility of obesity being linked to a disease.

Q. What's the Marine secret for slimming down?

A. Exercise is a major factor in slimming down. But Marines are taught that other critical factors are motivation and self-discipline. The conclusion is based on sound research. We know that when we eat more food than the body requires for our daily activities, the excess becomes body fat. This is true of all food—protein, carbohydrate and animal and vegetable fat. Throughout the Corps, whether the person is a recruit deliberately losing body fat or a general maintaining a lean physique, the rule is *eat less*. And that requires motivation and self-discipline.

Simply put, Marines establish the habit of eating less, until it becomes second nature to consume fewer calories. Marines also learn that exercise is useful in limiting overeating because a moderate workout curbs the appetite. As a result, a great many Marine men and women spend their lunch hour working out instead of eating out.

Q. How do you define excess body fat?

A. Based on the Marine minimum allowance, this would be anything over 18% for men and 26% for women. However, a lower goal may improve your performance and result in your feeling better.

Q. How long does it take to lose excess body fat?

A. Many recruits slim down in as little as 6 to 8 weeks. It's worth noting, however, that an overweight Marine is allowed up to 6 months to lose excess body fat. If the Marine succeeds in a partial but significant loss, an additional 6 months may be granted. This is based on the understanding that crash and quick-loss diets are counterproductive.